Alzheimer's Disease

Arun Jha • Kaushik Mukhopadhaya

Alzheimer's Disease

Diagnosis and Treatment Guide

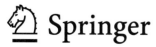 Springer

Arun Jha
Lambourn Grove Care Unit
Hertfordshire Partnership University NHS
Foundation Trust
St Albans
UK

Kaushik Mukhopadhaya
Hertfordshire Partnership University NHS
Foundation Trust
St Albans
UK

ISBN 978-3-030-56741-5   ISBN 978-3-030-56739-2   (eBook)
https://doi.org/10.1007/978-3-030-56739-2

This Springer imprint is published by the registered company Springer Nature Switzerland AG
The registered company address is: Gewerbestrasse 11, 6330 Cham, Switzerland

*To my esteemed teacher **Professor Mohan Mishra**, who taught me internal medicine in India in 1970s and inspired me to write this book by presenting his scientific paper on the clinical trial of herbal medicine for Alzheimer's disease in London in 2018, at the age of 80, with sincere thanks and debt of gratitude. I still use his techniques of neurological examination for differentiating Alzheimer's from vascular dementia.*

Arun Jha

*To my late father **Justice Suresh Chandra Mukherji** who taught me the values that made me the person I am and inspired me to serve humanity as a doctor.*

Kaushik Mukhopadhaya

Foreword

'The concept of treatable and untreatable dementias is no longer relevant; all dementias are treatable'. In this one sentence, Arun Jha and Kaushik Mukhopadhaya have set the tone of their discourse. Many believe that a good memory is the *sin qua non* of good cognition. This is OK as far as it goes, but memory itself is not a quantifiable commodity. What is memory after all and what are its types?

Memory acquisition consists of three stages—Recording, Retaining and Retrieving: you go to say a class room lecture, you try to record in your mind what have you heard and when you appear at the examination you attempt to retrieve what had you learnt and use it for your examination. You can use lecture notes for recording what have you learnt and use various ways of retaining information in your mind: mnemonics are popular wherein you use a word as a cue for remembering. This may work in a normal person but will not work in a person with dementia. Memory can be classified into long-term memory and short-term memory. This is easy enough, but you have to classify it into various types: these are implicit, explicit, episodic and semantic. These points are very beautifully tackled in the book by Jha and Mukhopadhaya. As a person ages, there is loss of memory and cognitive decline. Loss of memory is a normal process—as soon as you learn anything, you tend to forget it. So, you have to decide whether you really want to remember something in particular. As you grow old in age, you tend to forget many things which you would not if you were younger. Dementia is not confined to the old but occurs even in the relatively young.

Alzheimer is a syndrome in which there is cognitive decline beyond that expected of the patient's age. There are various types of dementia due to various causes; Alzheimer's is the commonest and the most important. The moment you make a diagnosis of Alzheimer's, you are faced with the question how long would the patient live and what course would the disease follow. Jha and Mukhopadhaya have produced a beautiful and well-structured book. Even if you are not a psychiatrist, you must have a copy of it. You may have to tackle this condition even in a non-specialist setting.

Darbhanga Medical College Hospital   Mohan Mishra
Bihar, India

Preface

Dementia due to Alzheimer's disease is a clinical syndrome causing disability and dependency among senior citizens worldwide, especially in low- and middle-income countries. It can be diagnosed and treated by all qualified doctors with little training and interest. While the underlying pathology is currently not reversible, the course of dementia might be modified with good care. The concept of treatable and non-treatable dementias is no longer relevant; all dementias are treatable. As the number of people with Alzheimer's dementia is rising, more and more frontline doctors in low-resource countries are expected to share the responsibility of its diagnosis and treatment. There is a wealth of new knowledge about the dementias stemming from advances in genetics, neuroscience, neuroimaging and changes in clinical approach. Many of the current available textbooks concentrate on basic sciences at the expense of practical advice; we have tried to avoid this trap by adopting a balanced approach. An unfamiliar reader would find this book a valuable guide in this rapidly advancing and fascinating field of medicine.

Primary care physicians are often expected to just get on with dementia assessment without a careful grounding in recent advances in Alzheimer's disease or how it should be applied to routine practice. Non-specialist doctors should find this guide particularly helpful as this book opens up areas that have traditionally been the province of the psychologist, psychiatrist and neurologist. There are chapters on neurobiology of cognition, taking clinical history and assessing cognition along with diagnosis and evidence-based treatment/care.

In 1917, the World Health Organization published the ***Global Action Plan*** *on the Public Response to Dementia 2017–2025* with seven action areas. The global target four states: '*In at least 50% of countries, as a minimum, 50% of the estimated number of people with dementia are diagnosed by 2025*'. Member states are expected to build the knowledge and skills of general and specialized staff in the health workforce to deliver evidence-based, culturally appropriate health and social care for people with dementia. This clinical guide is an attempt to contribute to achieving WHO global dementia action target of '*teaching health professionals the core competence of diagnosing and treating dementia due to Alzheimer's disease*'.

After the publication of the **WHO Dementia Report** in 2012, we got involved in establishing Alzheimer's and Related Dementias Society (ARDS) in Nepal. We have been contributing to the Nepalese dementia care by organizing teaching and training programmes for medical and nonmedical colleagues. There is a wide-held belief that only specialists can diagnose and treat dementia, and this has contributed to a fear of stepping out of line. The idea of this book was conceived when we were invited by the Nepalese Medical Association to organize an 'Alzheimer's Assessment' training workshop at its national conference in February 2020. The venue was Pokhara, a beautiful city at the foothill of snow-clad Annapurna mountain range. We could not resist the temptation to visit Pokhara, where one of us (AJ) had already done an 'Annapurna Memory Trek' a few years ago. It was like real homecoming. Preparation for the workshop sowed the seeds for gestation of this book. It should help our non-specialist colleagues venture into unchartered yet rewarding territory of dementia care.

This book is primarily aimed at front-line physicians in low- and middle-income countries, who have no previous experience of diagnosing and treating dementia. Developing clinical competence to deal with cognitive problems should help them care for older patients and their families in the developing world. To supplement this book, we have created an internet-based training organization, the *Memory First Aid International* (https://memoryfirstaid.uk), which would regularly provide learning materials for both medical and non-medical colleagues. Let us all join the '*Diagnose Dementia*' campaign across the world.

St Albans, UK   Arun Jha
St Albans, UK   Kaushik Mukhopadhaya

June 2020

"... Alzheimer's disease burdens an increasing number of our nation's elders and their families, and it is essential that we confront the challenges it poses to our public health ..."

President Barack Obama, *USA, 2011 (Quoted in WHO Dementia Report* 2012)

Acknowledgements

*Our sincere thanks to our colleague **Dr Michael Walker** at Hertfordshire Partnership University NHS Foundation Trust, for going through the draft manuscript and for providing valuable feedback to improve the quality and presentation of this book. We also sincerely thank our partners, **Meena** and **Neelanjana**, for their dedicated patience and encouragement in bringing this work to completion.*

*We thank **Melissa Morton**, the Executive Editor at Springer London, for guiding us from proposal to manuscript preparation to publication. Finally, we are grateful for our medical schoolteacher, **Professor Mohan Mishra**, for kindly agreeing to write the foreword for this book.*

Contents

About the Authors

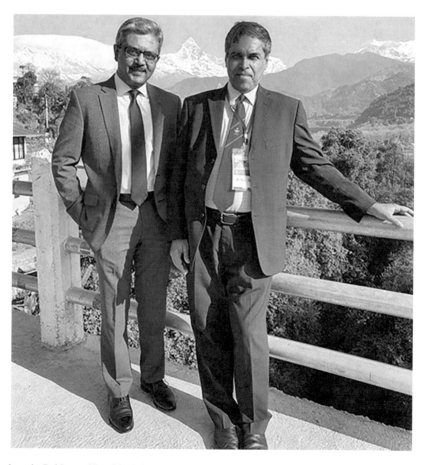

Authors in Pokhara, Nepal in February 2020 on the way to the Dementia Training organised by Nepalese Medical Association.

Chapter 1
Memory, Cognitive Impairment and Dementia

1.1 The First Meeting

At our NHS (UK National Health Service) specialist dementia diagnostic clinic (Memory Clinic), we have at least a 2 h slot for each new referral. We have been running such clinics since the publication of the National dementia strategy in 2009. Before seeing a patient, we have a series of documents and information at our disposal. The most important document is a referral letter from the patients' general practitioner (GP) outlining the reasons of the referral, summary of medical problems, list of current medications, and blood results. We also organise CT head scans for most patients and request an ECG from the GPs. Most GPs assess patients using a brief memory test, such as GPCOG. Half the job is already done.

In Hertfordshire, we run a joint assessment clinic with an experienced memory nurse, who takes a detailed history and conducts a basic daily-living assessment and a cognitive assessment using Addenbrooke's Cognitive Examination (ACE-III) [1] instrument. We also have access to a multidisciplinary team comprising of a clinical psychologist (for neuropsychological assessment, if and when required) and an occupational therapist for home functional assessment, if necessary. We follow NICE dementia assessment and treatment guidelines [2] at our specialist clinics. We are able make a diagnosis and agree a treatment plan in the vast majority of cases in one sitting. Patients and their family generally report their satisfaction. Apart from the frustration of increasing waiting time for initial assessment of over 12 weeks, there are very few complaints about the service. However, when we speak with our colleagues and relatives in our home countries (Nepal and India), we become acutely aware of the total lack of memory services there. These countries do not even have national dementia strategies in place, despite publication of WHO Dementia Report [3] in 2012.

As a front-line general physician in a non-specialist setting in Kathmandu, Kenya or Kent, when you see a patient in your clinic for the first time, you may not have

© The Editor(s) (if applicable) and The Author(s), under exclusive license to Springer Nature Switzerland AG 2021
A. Jha, K. Mukhopadhaya, *Alzheimer's Disease*,
https://doi.org/10.1007/978-3-030-56739-2_1

much information apart from their age and gender. The patient might have come for a routine blood pressure check or difficulty handling her new mobile phone. When, Dr. Alzheimer saw his first patient over a century ago, he was probably in a similar situation. He had no clue about his first patient (Box 1.1). At that time, people did not live long enough to develop late-life cognitive problems. He had probably never seen such an unusual patient with a bizarre combination of symptoms ever before (Box 1.1).

Box 1.1 Alzheimer's Eureka Moment 1 (A Patient with an Unusual Disease)

Alois Alzheimer (1864–1915) was a German psychiatrist and neuropathologist who observed a 51-year old patient Auguste Deter in 1901 whose sad story made her a household name throughout the world. He studied medicine in Berlin, Germany at a time when scientists were deepening their understanding of the effects of various diseases on the brain cells. Alzheimer's education had taught him the value of the microscope in exploring the causes and effects of disease. He wondered whether the same tool might be used in furthering the understanding of psychiatric disorders. After medical school, Alzheimer was able to follow up his ideas at a mental hospital in Frankfurt, where he was employed as a resident and subsequently as a senior physician.

In 1901, when Dr. Alzheimer met his world-famous patient, Auguste Deter (famous as "Auguste D"), he was a young psychiatrist in his late 30s, a hardworking clinician committed to understanding the relationship between brain disease and mental illness. Alzheimer was married in 1894 and had three children. After the tragic early death of his wife in 1901, Alzheimer moved to Heidelberg to join Emil Kraeplin in 1902. Subsequently, he moved to Munich in 1904. Following the death of his wife, he had submerged himself in his clinical work with psychiatric patients.

Auguste D was only 50 years old when her husband noticed her increasing memory problems. She soon became more fearful, paranoid, and aggressive, making it necessary to admit her to the psychiatric hospital at age 51. She remained an inpatient there until her death at the age of 55 in 1906. Alzheimer brought her medical records and post-mortem brain to Munich to work with new staining techniques in Emil Kraeplin's laboratory. One of Alzheimer's colleagues at the Munich laboratory was the famous Franz Nissl, who had developed special chemical stain for revealing structures within brain cells. In 1906, Alzheimer first described the clinical and pathological features of an *"unusual brain disease"* and published a short paper [4] in 1907. That famous case was later named with the eponym of 'Alzheimer's disease' by Kraeplin in 1910. Alzheimer had examined the patient's brain microscopically and found *'unusual things'* which are now called *plaques* and *tangles*. Alzheimer died at a young age of 51, as a result of a heart infection. His remains are buried in Frankfurt, next to those of his wife.

Such a case was never presented before. It was the careful mapping of the neuro-pathology of the brain of elderly people combined with attention to their clinical features prior to death that established Alzheimer's disease (AD) as the commonest cause of both young and late-onset dementia due to AD. AD became a disease entity, separate from normal ageing.

1.2 Introduction

Until recently there has been no '*test*' or '*treatment*' for Alzheimer's disease, (AD). No one believed that AD could be prevented. But remarkable progress has been made in past few decades, especially since the first drug, *donepezil*, was introduced in 1997. Many of dementia's manifestations are known to be manageable. While the underlying illness is not curable, the course might be modified. Available interventions and care can improve the trajectory of symptoms and the family's ability to cope with them. Evidence for prevention is also emerging.

In 2017, the *Lancet* launched a Commission [5] to review the available evidence and produced recommendations about how best to manage and prevent dementia. This is perhaps one of the best scientific papers on dementia published in recent years and is a must-read for every dementia care clinician. Although the symptoms of AD generally occur in later life, the underlying brain pathology develops many years earlier. Alzheimer's disease is a clinically silent disorder that begins in midlife (about age 40–65 years) and the terminal stage manifests as symptoms of dementia. It is rightly said that, *AD is an illness of midlife that manifests in later life*. The key messages (five out of ten) of the Lancet Commission include (1) Treat cognitive symptoms; (2) Individualise dementia care; (3) Care for family carers; (4) Plan for the future; (Manage neuropsychiatric symptoms. These messages accord the WHO Global Action Plan on the public health Response to Dementia (2017–2025) [6]. Diagnosis of dementia is often delayed due to the mistaken belief that dementia is a natural consequence of ageing or because of an individual's reluctance to seek help about their memory problems or lack of competence and confidence among front-line physicians, especially in developing countries, to diagnose and treat dementia in early stages.

Many national and international guidelines recommend that people with suspected dementia are referred to a specialist memory clinic or individual specialist doctor for diagnosis and treatment. These guidelines recommend a systematic approach, including history taking from the patient and informant, blood tests, and structured cognitive assessment. However, specialist dementia diagnosis services are not available in most low and middle-income countries. Consequently, it is often families or unskilled friends who try to manage the initial problems associated with dementia, without having any awareness of the underlying diagnosis.

Failing to recognise dementia can cause difficulties for people with dementia and for their families who generally have no understanding of the changes taking place. This ignorance may lead to neglect and abuse. To improve the recognition and diagnosis of early dementia General physicians and primary health care professionals require education and training. The key management tasks in early dementia of any aetiology are helping the patient and family come to terms with the diagnosis, maximise quality of life in the present, and planning for the future. This clinical guide for health professionals aims to do just that.

1.3   What Is Normal?

It is normal to have occasional memory lapses and to lose things. It is normal to forget why we have gone upstairs, or to come back from a shopping trip without the very thing we went for. It is normal to have to search our brain for a name, sometimes. Our normal memory may suffer, from time to time, from impaired function through inattention, information overload or mild depression. Unless there is something wrong, we retain a huge store of general knowledge (semantic) an ability to plan and manage our affairs and, under normal circumstances anyway, we retain our orientation in time and place.

> **Cognition** is defined as the mental processes used to obtain knowledge or to become aware of and interact with the environment. These processes include perception, imagination, judgement, memory, and language.

Cognitive abilities can be divided into several specific cognitive domains; these are attention, memory, executive cognitive function, language, and visuospatial abilities.

For diagnostic purpose, the *Diagnostic and Statistical Manual of Me*ntal *Disorders, 5th Edition* [7] (DSM-5 defines **six key domains** of cognitive function—*complex attention, executive function, learning* and *memory, language, perceptual-motor ability,* and *social cognition.* Box 1.2 provides definitions and examples of these terms as described in DSM-5.

> **Box 1.2 Cognitive Domains Defined in DSM-5 Neurocognitive Disorder**
> *Major neurocognitive disorder* (what is generally known as dementia) *is an acquired disorder with significant cognitive decline in one or more of the following domains:*
>
> - *Complex attention* (sustained attention, selective attention, processing speed). Example deficits: difficulty with multiple stimuli, easily distracted, unable to perform mental calculations.

- *Executive function* (planning, decision making, working memory, responding to feedback/error correction, overriding habits, mental flexibility). Example deficits: unable to do complex projects, extra effort required to organise, social gatherings reported as taxing.
- *Learning and memory* (immediate memory, recent memory (including free recall, cued recall, and recognition memory), very long-term memory. Example deficits: repeats self in conversation, can't keep a shopping list, requires frequent reminders.
- *Language* (expressive language [including naming, fluency, and grammar and syntax] and receptive language). Example deficits: using general phrases ("that thing on your foot") rather than the name of an object ("shoe"), trouble with names of family members, grammatical errors.
- *Perceptual-motor ability* (construction and visual perception, perceptual-motor, praxis, gnosis). Example deficits: trouble with previous familiar activities, trouble navigating familiar environments, trouble with spatial tasks.
- *Social cognition* (recognition of emotions, theory of mind, behaviour regulation). Example deficits: behaviour out of acceptable social range, insensitivity to social standards, makes decisions without regard to safety.

For each of these domains, a person must first perceive the stimulus, process the information, and then respond. Both sensory perception and processing of speed decline with age, thus impacting test performance in many cognitive domains. For example, hearing begins to decline after age 30, and up to 70% of people aged 80 have measurable hearing loss. Also, speech discrimination and sound localisation decrease with advancing age. Additionally, there is a clear decline in processing speed, making older people perform cognitive abilities more slowly than younger adults.

1.4   Memory

The human brain has the remarkable capacity to acquire, store, and recall information across decades of time. **Learning** is the acquisition of new information or skills. **Memory** is the retention of learned material. Remembering consists of three stages:

1. *Acquisition* or *encoding* is learning the material
2. *Storage* is keeping the information until it is needed, and
3. *Retrieval* is finding the material and getting it back out when required

"Three R's of Remembering" can help us remember these three stages, corresponding with **R**ecording (acquisition), **R**etaining (storage), and **R**etrieving (Fig. 1.1).

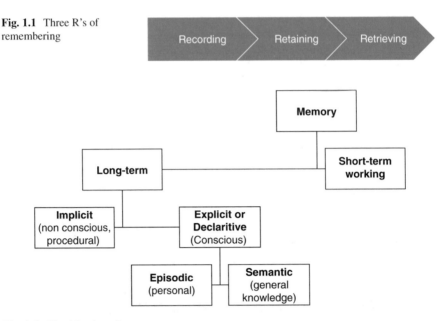

Fig. 1.1 Three R's of remembering

Fig. 1.2 Classification of memory

   Most problems in remembering come at the retrieval rather than storage stage. We are all very aware that memory is limited more in getting things out than getting them in. More can be stored in memory than can be retrieved. There is not much we can do to improve retrieval directly, but retrieval is a function of how the material is recorded and retained. Therefore, improved methods of recording and retaining will improve retrieval. People with mild memory problems can be trained to record and retain information in such a way as to be able to retrieve it more effectively.

   A useful framework for assessing memory impairment is to divide it into separate memory systems—*Long* and *Short-term*, and domains—*episodic* memory, *semantic* memory and *working* memory (Fig. 1.2). Memory of facts and events is called **declarative or explicit memory**. A declarative *Episodic memory* consists of autobiographical (personally experienced events). The basic features of episodic memory are summarised in Box 1.3.

Box 1.3 Features of Episodic Memory
- *The memory content is consciously available for access, and can be expressed verbally or by other means, such as drawing, and*
- *The memory trace pertains to an experienced past event*
- *It depends on the integrity of the medial temporal lobes*
- *Episodic memory impairment is usually the first cognitive symptom of AD*

Semantic (conceptual) memory involves memory for word meaning facts and general knowledge. Explicit or declarative memory is what people usually mean in everyday uses of the word "memory". Episodic memory matters are unique to the individual, e.g. what they ate for breakfast, and depends on an intact hippocampus.

Generally, declarative memories are accessed for conscious recollection, whereas the tasks we learn, as well as the reflexes and emotional associations we have formed, operate smoothly without conscious recollection. For example, we may not explicitly remember the day we first rode a bike on our own (the declarative part of the memory), but our brain remembers what to do when we are on the bike (the procedural part of the memory). Another feature of declarative memories is that they are easy to form and are easily forgotten. In contrast, forming implicit (nondeclarative) memories usually require repetition and practice over a longer period of time, but these memories are less likely to be forgotten. While there is no clear limit to the number of declarative memories the brain can store, there is great diversity in the ease and speed with which such new information is acquired.

1.4.1 Long-and Short-Term Memory

Some memories last longer than others. *Long-term memories* are those that you can recall days, months, or years after they were originally stored. Most information, however, is held by the brain only temporarily, generally for a few hours. These **short-term memories** are vulnerable to disruption. Learning and memory can be considered as occurring in two stages: *acquisition* and *consolidation*. Memory **acquisition** (learning) occurs by a *physical modification of the brain* caused by incoming sensory information. This is different from working memory, which is vulnerable to erasure by distraction and this has very limited capacity (think about holding a phone number in mind). Working memory can be achieved by keeping neural activity going with continuous rehearsal and does not require any lasting physical change in the brain. In contrast, short-term memory survives distraction, has a larger capacity, and can last minutes to hours with no conscious effort. These memories persist for some time without rehearsal but are considered to be 'short-term' because they will be forgotten unless they are consolidated into long-term memory. **Consolidation** is the process by which some experiences, held temporarily by transient modifications of neurones, are selected for permanent storage in long-term memory (Fig. 1.3).

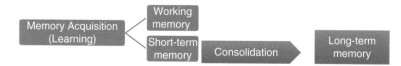

Fig. 1.3 Memory consolidation

When someone tells you his or her phone number, you can retain it for a limited period of time by repeating the number to yourself. Keeping a memory alive through repetition or rehearsal is a hallmark of another type of memory called **working memory**. Unlike the short-term memory, working memories are sharply limited in capacity. It is said that working memory is information held "in mind". If the number is too long (e.g., a phone number with an area code), you may have trouble remembering the number at all. Working memory is commonly assessed by examining a person's *digit span*, the maximum number of randomly chosen numbers a person can repeat back after hearing a list read. The normal digit span is 7 plus or minus 2. Working memory is distinguished from short-term memory by the very limited capacity, the need for repetition, and the very short duration.

Information held in working memory might be converted into long-term memories, but most of it is discarded when no longer needed. How is information retained in the brain by working memory long enough to be useful? Recent research suggests that the rostral end of the frontal lobe, the **prefrontal cortex**, which is very well developed in humans, is involved in higher mental functions such as *self-awareness*, complex *planning*, *judgement* and p*roblem solving*.

1.4.2   Measures of Memory

There are three main ways to measure how much a person remembers. We can ask him to tell us everything he remembers; we can ask him to pick out the items he remembers from a group of items; or we can see how easily he learns the material a second time. These three approaches are referred to, respectively, as *recall, recognition,* and *relearning.*

Recall requires producing information by searching the memory for it. When most people say they do not remember something, what they mean is that they do not recall it. A person who is unable to recall something may be able to recall it if he is given some cues. This is called *cued* or *aided recall.* On the other hand, in the *free-recall* method a person is presented a list of words one at a time and required to learn the list so that he can recall as many words as possible in any order. An example of free recall in everyday life is remembering the items on a shopping list. In the *paired-associate* method, pairs of words are shown, and the person is required to associate them so that when he is given the first word, he will recall the second word. Learning the capitals of countries is an example of this method.

Recognition—a person may be unable to recall something even when given cues but may still show evidence of remembering if recognition is used as the measure of memory. The word *recognition* means literally "to know again". *When* we recognise something, we acknowledge that it is familiar, that we have met it before.

In recognition the test is, 'is this the item?"; in recall the test is, "what is the item?" An example of a recognition task in examination is a multiple-choice question. Recognition is usually easier than recall because we do not have to search for the information; it is given to us and all we have to do is be able to identify it as something we learned. Although most older adults do not perform as well as most young adults in free-recall tasks, they do perform well in recognition or cued-recall tasks. Most people remember other people's faces better than their names. One reason is that remembering a face is usually a recognition task and remembering a name is usually a recall task. Generally speaking, we are more concerned with recall than with recognition because most of us have the greatest problem with recall. In Alzheimer's disease, patients can lose both recall and recognition abilities.

1.4.3 How and Why We Forget?

Learning new information alters the physiological state of certain neurones that encode memory. These state changes, or molecular and cellular and memory traces, can be any change in the activity of the cell that is induced by the learning that becomes part of the neural code of that memory. Neuroscientists call these memory traces 'engram' [8]. Acquisition leads to short-term memories that persist for seconds or minutes, intermediate-term memories that last for a few hours, and long-term memory that can persist for years or decades.

An early declarative memory might be encoded by a group of hippocampal neurones, but the engram become distributed to other brain regions through the process of consolidation. Although forgetting can occur due to a failed retrieval of an intact engram, active forgetting seems to happen through the biological degradation of molecular and cellular circuits. This would make the memory engram incomplete and unresponsive to recall mechanisms.

The brain has the inherent capacity to erase memories through psychological and biological mechanisms. There are several psychological theories to explain why we forget. Psychologists usually provide five common explanations [9]:

- *Decay.* This explanation suggests that the memory trace "engram" in the brain decays or fades away with time. The basis of forgetting is disuse.
- *Repression.* This is the psychodynamic explanation suggested by Sigmund Freud on the unconscious mind, when unpleasant or unacceptable memories are pushed back (repressed) into subconscious chamber of the mind. This is a defence mechanism used so that the person will not have to live with them.
- *Distortion.* Memories may be affected by our values and interests, so that we remember somethings the way we *want* to remember them. This explanation suggests that we change our memories to fit with what we want them to be or how we feel they should be.
- *Interference.* Forgetting might takes place due to interference by other learning. For instance, one might fail to retrieve on a particular day the location of one's car in the parking lot used daily due to competition from similar memory traces accumulated across the prior month. There is no clear active process underlying this failure of memory retrieval; it is rather passive in nature. However, competing memories formed shortly before or after acquisition of another may interfere

actively with memory storage discussed above. Thus, forgetting through interference mechanisms can be viewed as both passive and active depending on when the interfering material was learned and whether it maintains or erodes memory traces.

- *Cue dependency.* Recent research suggests that some memory trace (engram) remains sufficiently intact across time to be constituted by a brief reminder or a cue, despite the apparent loss of memory without a reminder. Waiting for a longer period before testing the memory may deteriorate the engram further so that a cue no longer strengthens it. This explanation is referred to as "cue-dependent forgetting."

1.4.4   How Fast Do We Forget?

Even across a single day, the brain is bombarded with new information that increases excitatory process for learning. Forgetting can be viewed as an 'intrinsic' homeostatic mechanism to bring the brain back to its basal state. It operates continuously at a low level to slowly remove each newly acquired memory. Consolidation would play the role of the judge, allowing memories that are deemed important and worthwhile to remain while allowing the irrelevant ones removed by intrinsic forgetting.

Research indicates that the clearance of irrelevant memories opens new storage space and facilitates retrieval, making the brain more efficient for error-free retrieval. The neuronal circuits that promote forgetting are regulated by external factors and internal states, including activity, stress, and sleep. Sleep enhances memory consolidation and inhibit active forgetting.

Active forgetting, along with attention, acquisition, and consolidation are the brains biological system for managing memories. Deficits in active forgetting may be the pathophysiology of Alzheimer's and other brain disorders. Research is underway to identify molecular targets for cognitive enhancers.

1.4.5   Ageing and Memory

As we get older, we become annoyed at ourselves as it becomes increasingly hard to remember to post a letter or where we put our car keys. Many people begin to worry quite seriously at this stage, seeing this forgetfulness not just as a sign of ageing, but as a possible indication of Alzheimer's disease. In actual fact, the patterns of memory loss are different.

For most of us, the problem is not the memory has been wiped clean, but that we experience difficulty in retrieving it. Given the right cues, or even equipped with our own methods of remembering, we can come up with the right answer. Research has indicated that older people can perform just as well as younger counterparts in memory and cognitive tests, but they respond better to comfortable conditions and a relaxed schedule. Given the pressure of time and stress in the environment, their ability becomes impaired.

Memory problems are not a definite sign of dementia. In fact, statistics indicate that only 10–15% of the population develop Alzheimer's disease, and its effects on the memory are different and unmistakable. People with normal age-related memory loss tend to experience an increase in those 'tip of the tongue' memory moments, where they know they know something, but cannot quite recall it—usually because it is not an item, they need to recall every day. People with Alzheimer's disease, in contrast, forget the names and functions of objects they encounter in their daily lives.

It was once believed that we are born with finite number of neurones, and that from birth this declines. Nowadays it is understood that the actual volume of tissue lost due to ageing is very small. What does suffer significant loss is the *basal forebrain*, the area that supplies acetylcholine to the hippocampus. It is argued that this affects the plasticity of the brain, making it increasingly hard for the brain of an older person to adapt to changing circumstances. A key protein called *PPI*, seems to have a role in deleting memories. By blocking its action, researchers found that they could boost the learning and memory capacities of mice.

1.4.5.1 Amnesia

In daily life, forgetting happens as often as learning. Certain diseases and brain injuries cause a serious loss of memory and/or the ability to learn called **amnesia**. Concussion, chronic alcoholism, encephalitis, brain tumour, stroke and Alzheimer's disease can all disrupt memory.

Some patients try to fill up the gaps in their memory by creating false memories. *Confabulation* is the confident recounting of 'false memories' for recent events. For example, a patient with no memory of what they ate for breakfast may confabulate a completely incorrect menu. This is done in a plausible manner without any apparent difficulty, and without any awareness of the falsity of the information. Confabulation is common in Alzheimer's disease and in alcoholic amnestic syndrome.

Following trauma to the brain, two different types of memory loss may occur: retrograde amnesia and anterograde amnesia. **Retrograde amnesia** is characterised by memory loss for events prior to the brain injury; you forget things you already knew. **Anterograde amnesia** is an inability to form new memories following brain trauma. In clinical cases, there is often a mixture of retrograde and anterograde amnesia of different degrees of severity.

Retention of newly learned information is relatively stable with advancing age, but retrieval of information may require more cueing or a recognition format to remain stable in advanced age groups. Prospective memory, specifically remembering to perform intended action in the future (e.g., taking medication after breakfast), declines with age. Procedural memories, such as remembering how to play or ride a bike, are preserved with age.

1.4.5.2 Memory and Hippocampus

Memory formation, retention and retrieval involve a system of interconnected brain areas. The medial temporal lobe, especially the **hippocampus**, seems essential for declarative memory. The hippocampus plays a crucial role in *binding* sensory information for the purpose of memory consolidation. It also supports *spatial* memory of the location of objects of behavioural importance. Finally, the hippocampus is involved in the *storage* of memories for some length of time.

1.4.6 Biological Ageing

The shrinkage of the cerebral cortex and the loss of synaptic density appear to begin in early adulthood, and both follow a linear trajectory of decline across the lifespan into old age and yet cognition is not affected at this early age. Within the brain the passage of time is not only associated with the downward trajectory of biological ageing, but also the upward trajectory of learning from experience. In general, it appears that the elderly brain does become slower to learn but it never loses the capacity to learn. Also, information and skills learnt throughout life appear resilient to old age. There is, however, a loss of intellectual speed and flexibility which is observed even amongst the 'super-elderly', that is, very intelligent elderly people in very good health. This suggests that everyone experiences some loss of cognitive power in old age but that usually the cognitive decline is mild and the impact of such decline on everyday life is minimal.

The extent to which biological ageing and the age-related diseases are truly separable remains controversial. The progressive nature of dementing conditions makes it extremely difficult to distinguish between the earliest signs of a neurodegenerative process and the normal effects of brain ageing. There appears to be no pathological or physiological marker that clearly distinguishes between elderly people with and without dementia. According to the *continuum hypothesis* 'normal ageing' and 'dementia' are seen as lying along a continuum of cognitive decline in old age, ranging from the very mild decline experienced by the 'super-elderly' through to the catastrophic declines associated with severe dementia. With Alzheimer's disease being the dominant cause of dementia, and with age being the dominant risk factor for this condition, the continuum model of dementia is often viewed as being interchangeable with the question, "Is Alzheimer's disease a true disease or accelerated ageing?". This is an over-simplistic and misleading question. Other dementias which are not caused by Alzheimer's are not considered to be the same disease. If, not all dementias are caused by Alzheimer's, then it is most unlikely that all 'normal ageing' is caused by Alzheimer's disease. The *multifactorial theory* suggests that the decline of cognition in extreme old age is associated with the accumulation of several mild and separate (distinct) challenges to the brain, rather than the intensification of a single process.

A variety of factors can cause cumulative damage to the brain with age and produce cognitive impairments. These factors include damage to the brain due to cerebral ischaemia, head injuries, toxins such as alcohol, excess stress hormones, or development of degenerative diseases such as Alzheimer's disease.

1.5   What Is Dementia?

The word dementia is derived from the Latin words *de* (out of) and *mens* (mind). Dementia is the most feared illness in people over the age of 55. The brain is the organ that we least understand. We don't just fear the loss of memory—in a very real way, we fear the loss of who we are. Dementia has been renamed *Major Neurocognitive Disorder*. The new terminology has been selected in part to avoid the stigma associated with the word *dementia* when categorising deficits among younger people with progressive cognitive decline, such as that associated with HIV infection or traumatic brain injury. Neurocognitive disorders have cognitive impairment as their presenting problem, rather than disorders that are congenital or apparent in childhood (most importantly in contrast to learning disability). They may be secondary (i.e. those attributed to medical conditions or the effects of drugs) or primary and *degenerative* (i.e., those that reflect a decline from a previously attained level of cognitive functioning). Disorders in this category include *delirium, major neurocognitive disorders,* and *mild neurocognitive* disorders, and are attributable to changes in brain structure, function, or chemistry.

Dementia is a syndrome—usually of a chronic or progressive nature—in which there is deterioration in cognitive function (i.e. the ability to process thought) beyond what might be expected from normal ageing. It affects memory, thinking, orientation, comprehension, calculation, learning capacity, language, and judgement. Consciousness is not affected. The cognitive impairment is commonly accompanied by deterioration in emotional control, social behaviour, or motivation.

Dementia results from a variety of diseases and injuries affecting the brain, such as Alzheimer's disease or stroke. Dementia due to Alzheimer's disease is the most common type, contributing up to 70% of cases. It can be overwhelming, not only for the person who has it, but also for their family and relatives. There is often a lack of awareness and understanding of Alzheimer's, resulting in stigmatisation and barriers to diagnosis and care.

Worldwide, around 50 million people have dementia, with nearly 60% living in low- and middle-income countries. Every year, there are nearly ten million new cases. This figure translates into *one new case every 3* s. Most new case (71%) are expected to occur in low- and middle-income countries. The estimated prevalence of dementia in the elderly population aged 60 and over is between 5 and 8%.

Dementia leads to increased cost for governments, communities, families and individuals, and to loss in productivity for economies. In 2020, the total global societal cost of dementia was estimated to be over 1.1% of global gross domestic product (GDP).

There are many different causes and types of dementia (Box 1.4). Primary dementias include dementia due to Alzheimer's disease (AD), vascular dementia, dementia with Lewy bodies and frontotemporal dementia. AD is the most common, followed by vascular dementia and dementia with Lewy bodies. Mixed dementia with features of more than one type is also common, especially in older adults. For the scope of this clinical guide, we will discuss only dementia due to Alzheimer's disease or Alzheimer's dementia (AD).

Box 1.4 WHO New Classification of Dementia [10]

- *Dementia due to Alzheimer's disease*
- *Dementia due to cerebrovascular disease*
- *Dementia due to Lewy body disease*
- *Dementia due to use of alcohol*
- *Dementia due to use of sedatives, hypnotics or anxiolytics*
- *Dementia due to use of volatile inhalants*
- *Dementia due to Parkinson's disease*
- *Dementia due to exposure to heavy metals and other toxins*
- *Dementia due to HIV*
- *Dementia due to multiple sclerosis*
- *Dementia due to prion disease*
- *Dementia due to normal pressure hydrocephalus*
- *Dementia due to injury to the head*
- *Dementia due to pellagra*
- *Dementia due to Down's syndrome*
- *Dementia due to other specified diseases classified elsewhere*

1.5.1 Why Should Dementia Be Identified Early?

There are arguments for early diagnosis but, for a variable condition with an insidious onset and a slow prodrome, such as dementia, the earlier the diagnosis is attempted the harder it is to be sure about it. On the other hand, there are compelling arguments against delaying or avoiding diagnosis: medication does help many people to become '*more themselves*' for a useful period of time. There is thus an opportunity for individuals and families to maximise enjoyable activities and plan to mitigate potential difficulties or crises. Globally, public awareness of dementia has generally improved, but not sufficiently.

We are moving away from the concept of protecting patients from the diagnosis because 'nothing can be done', and towards offering 'timely' diagnosis to patients. This means that diagnosis need to be linked to any particular stage of dementia, and that people and families can be enabled to access the support when they need it. We should respect the decision of patients and families to present themselves at a time that is right for them.

A large-scale cross-sectional online survey [11] of primary care physicians and specialists across five European countries, Canada, and the USA revealed current clinical practices and barriers related to the diagnostic process for patients presenting with suspected MCI or AD. Participants were asked to identify barriers to prompt diagnosis from prespecified lists of known diagnostic challenges, categorised into four domains: patient-related, physician-related, setting-related, and those relating to the clinical profile of AD.

Physicians reported a range of barriers when attempting to diagnose MCI and AD. Major themes included patients seeing cognitive decline as a normal part of ageing and not disclosing symptoms, long waiting lists, and lack of treatment options and definitive biomarker tests. Primary care physicians identified burdens on the healthcare system, such as *long waiting lists and inadequate time to evaluate patients*. Some of the physician-related barriers are listed in Box 1.5.

Box 1.5 Physician-Related Barriers of Diagnosis
- Impact of diagnosis on the patient (37%)
- Struggle to identify when cognitive impairment is not present due to normal ageing (32%)
- Consequences of an inaccurate diagnosis (30%)
- Primary care physicians were more likely than specialists to indicate that they had inadequate training to diagnose AD (20% vs. 8%)

If 20% of primary care physicians in European and north American countries indicate lack of adequate knowledge to diagnose AD, it is easy to infer that a vast majority of physicians in the low and middle-income countries may feel completely out of depth. These findings are useful for identifying target audiences for interventions intended to improve their diagnostic capability.

1.5.2 Prevalence of Dementia in South Asian Countries

The prevalence of clinically diagnosed AD increases exponentially with age. *At age 65, less than 5% of the population has clinical AD, but the number increases to more than 40% beyond age 85.* The Alzheimer's Disease International Report [12] 2014 provides estimated number of people with dementia (Table 1.1) in the Asia Pacific region consisting of 18 ADI member Associations in Australia, Bangladesh, China, Taipei, Hong Kong, India, Indonesia, Japan, Macau, Malaysia, Nepal, New Zealand, Pakistan, Philippines, Singapore, Republic of Korea, Sri Lanka and Thailand. The number of people with dementia in Nepal, for example, is estimated to increase from **78,000** in 2015 to **134,000** by 2030, and **285,000** by 2050.

Table 1.1 Projected prevalence of dementia in South Asian countries from 2015–2050

	Projected population (million)	Estimated number of people with dementia ('000)		
	Y2015	Y2015	Y2030	Y2050
ADI members				
Bangladesh	160,411	460	834	1193
China	1,401,587	10,590	18,116	32,184
India	1,282,390	4031	6743	12,542
Nepal	28,441	78	134	285
Pakistan	188,144	450	712	1422
Sri Lanka	21,612	147	262	463

1.5.3   Risk Factors for Alzheimer's Dementia

Of all the risk factors for AD, age is the most important, doubling the risk every 5 years after the age of 65. Overall, about 80% of cases of dementia are in people aged 75 years or older. There is an interaction between age, neuropathology, comorbidities and the clinical presentation. Age on its own is a less powerful risk factor once other risk factors and comorbidities are taken into account, none the less it still remains an important consideration, especially as life expectancy continues to increase.

There is an element of inheritance as there is an interesting interaction between age and genetic factors. The only confirmed genetic risk factor, *APOE* (Box 1.6), alters the age of onset rather than having an absolute risk of developing the condition.

Box 1.6 APOE Gene (Source: National Institute of Health [7])
Apolipoprotein E (ApoE) is a major cholesterol carrier that supports lipid transport and injury repair in the brain. The *APOE* gene provides instructions for making a protein called apolipoprotein E. This protein combines with lipids in the body to form molecules called lipoproteins. Lipoproteins are responsible for packaging cholesterol and other fats and carrying them through the blood stream. Maintaining normal levels of cholesterol is essential for the prevention of cardiovascular diseases, including heart attack and stroke. There are at least three slightly different versions (alleles) of the *APOE* gene. The major alleles are called e2, e3, and e4. The most common allele is e3, which is found in more than half of the general population.

Individuals carrying the e4 allele are at increased risk of AD (both early and late onset) compared with those carrying the more common e3 allele, whereas the e2 allele decreases risk. Presence of APOEe4 allele is also associated with increased risk for cerebral amyloid angiopathy and age-related cognitive decline during normal ageing.

1.5.3.1 Modifiable Risk Factors

Dementia is heterogeneous and risk factors vary, and often coexist, for different types of dementia. Some dementia risk factors, including cardiovascular disease, cerebrovascular disease, metabolic and psychiatric factors, diet, lifestyle, and education, are potentially modifiable. Vascular brain injury, for instance, not only leads to vascular dementia, but also occurs more commonly in older people with AD than those without AD and is present in some people who do not have dementia. It is possible to influence potentially modifiable risk factors and prevent or delay onset of dementia to some extent.

1.5.4 Inside Alzheimer's Brain [13]

Many molecular and cellular changes take place in the brain of a person with AD.

The most important change is the deposition of two abnormal proteins: *Amyloid Plaques* (Box 1.7) and *Neurofibrillary tangles (NFTs)*. Amyloid makes sticky plaques in the brain while tau forms tangles as the nerve cells are damaged with the progress of the disease.

Box 1.7 AD Eureka Moment 2 (Plaques and Tangles) [13]
In 1984, the identification of the beta-amyloid protein in the blood vessels of patients with Down's syndrome and Alzheimer's disease suggested that the 21st chromosome (present as an extra copy in people with Down's syndrome) might hold clues to understanding AD pathology. This proved true when beta amyloid was identified in 1987 as an important component of senile plaques and was linked to a gene located on chromosome 21. Soon after, in the early 1990s, the discovery of gene mutations prompted the "amyloid cascade" hypothesis. According to this hypothesis 'AD pathology results from accumulation of amyloid plaques in the brain leading to an inflammatory response and brain cell death'.

The beta-amyloid protein involved in AD comes in several different forms that collect between neurones. It is formed from the breakdown of a larger protein, called *amyloid precursor protein*. One form, **beta-amyloid 42**, is thought to be especially toxic. In AD brain, abnormal levels of this naturally occurring protein clump together to form plaques that collect between neurones and disrupt cell function.

Two years later, tangles of tau protein were also discovered in patients with Alzheimer's disease. Plaques and tangles cause brain cell damage.

Neurofibrillary Tangles (NFTs) are abnormal accumulation of protein called *tau* that collect inside neurones. Normally, healthy neurones are supported internally by structures called *microtubules* that help guide nutrients and molecules from the cell body to the axon and dendrites. In healthy neurones, tau normally binds to and stabilises microtubules. In AD, abnormal chemical changes cause tau to detach from microtubules and stick to other tau molecules, forming threads that eventually join to form tangles inside neurones. These insoluble twisted fibres (tangles) found inside the brain cells block the neuronal transport system, which harms the synaptic communication between neurones.

The exact mechanism involved in Alzheimer's brain changes is not known. Emerging evidence suggests that Alzheimer's-related brain changes may result from a complex interplay among abnormal **tau** and **beta-amyloid** proteins and several other factors.

1.6   Preventing Alzheimer's by Active Ageing

Until a few years ago, prevention of dementia seemed like wishful thinking, but now there is some emerging evidence to suggest that keeping vascular risk factors under control is always worthwhile, as is keeping weight down and exercising. Keeping mentally active and retaining social networks is also good. There is no hard evidence for vitamins in preventing dementia.

Active ageing is key to successful ageing. Active ageing involves the optimisation of psychosocial interventions. It is important to recognise that promoting active ageing is preventing illness and disability and increasing wellbeing in old age. There are many studies that demonstrate that physical activity is prerequisite for successful ageing. A young but physically inactive individual seems old, just as an old but active individual appears young. Physical activity also has positive effects on psychological wellbeing by promoting mental abilities, subjective wellbeing, social skills, and self-concept.

Cognitive activity is equally important for successful ageing. Many studies have found that mentally active individuals who have a wide range of interests, and a large number of social contacts greater psycho-physical wellbeing than those who lack such activity. Research supports that there is broad cognitive plasticity and reserve capacity throughout the lifecycle including old age. Cognitive training can compensate cognitive decline in healthy elderly. Even people with MCI and mild AD show cognitive plasticity to some extent.

Two recent guidelines are extremely important in dementia care—*Lancet guideline 12017* [3] and *WHO guidelines 2019* [4]. Dementia syndrome is heterogenous and some risk factors are modifiable. Around 35% of dementia is attributable to a combination of nine risk factors (Table 1.2)

Although age is the strongest risk factor for dementia, it is not an inevitable consequence of ageing. People can reduce their risk of developing dementia, especially Alzheimer's and vascular types, by getting regular exercise, not smoking, avoiding

Table 1.2   Potentially modifiable risk factors for dementia [3]

Early life (age <18 years Less education (none or primary school only)	Relative risk of dementia 1.6	Prevalence 40%
Midlife (age 45–65 years)		
Hypertension	1.6	8.9%
Obesity	1.6	3.4%
Hearing loss	1.9	31.7%
Late life (age >65 years)		
Smoking	1.6	27.4%
Depression	1.9	13.2%
Physical inactivity	1.4	17.7%
Social isolation	1.6	11.0%
Diabetes	1.5	06.4%

harmful use of alcohol, controlling their weight, eating healthy diet, and maintaining healthy blood pressure, cholesterol and blood sugar levels.

Among the vascular risk factors, hypertension tops the list. Obesity is linked to pre-diabetes and metabolic syndrome, which is characterised by insulin resistance and high concentrations of peripheral insulin. Peripheral insulin anomalies are thought to cause a decrease in brain insulin production, which can impair amyloid clearance. An increase in inflammation and high blood glucose concentrations could also be mechanisms by which diabetes impairs cognition.

1.6.1   WHO Dementia Risk Reduction Guideline

Certain medical conditions are associated with an increased risk of developing dementia, including hypertension, diabetes, hypercholesterolaemia, obesity and depression. In May 2017, WHO endorsed the *Global Action Plan on the Public Health Response to Dementia 2017–2025* [4]. The action plan includes seven strategic action areas and dementia risk reduction is one of them. Based on the emerging evidence, WHO has issued specific dementia risk prevention guideline (Box 1.8).

Box 1.8 WHO Dementia Risk Reduction Guideline 2019 [4]
- *Physical activity* should be recommended to adults with normal cognition to reduce the risk of cognitive decline
- *Interventions for tobacco cessation* should be offered to adults who use tobacco since they may reduce the risk of cognitive decline and dementia in addition to other health benefits
- *A healthy, balanced diet* should be recommended to all adults based on WHO recommendations on healthy diet

- *Interventions for alcohol use disorders* should be offered to adults with normal cognition and mild cognitive impairment to reduce the risk of cognitive decline and/or dementia in addition to other health benefits
- *Management of hypertension* should be offered to adults with hypertension according to existing WHO guidelines
- *The management of diabetes* in the form of medications and/or lifestyle interventions should be offered to adults with diabetes
- *Management of dyslipidaemia at mid-life may be offered to reduce the risk of cognitive decline and dementia*

References

1. Hodges JR, Larner AJ. Cognitive screening instruments: a practical approach. In: Addenbrooke's cognitive examinations: ACE, ACE-R, ACE-III, ACE app, and M-ACE. 2nd ed. Berlin: Springer; 2017. p. 109–37.
2. https://www.nice.org.uk/guidance/ng97
3. https://www.who.int/mental_health/publications/dementia_report_2012/en/
4. Cipriani G, Dolciotti C, Picchi L, et al. Alzheimer and his disease: a brief history. Neurol Sci. 2011;32:275.
5. Livingston G, Sommerlad A, Orgeta V, et al. Dementia prevention, intervention, and care. Lancet. 2017;390:2673–734.
6. https://www.who.int/mental_health/neurology/dementia/action_plan_2017_2025/en/
7. American Psychiatric Association, editor. Diagnostic and statistical manual of mental disorders. 5th ed. Washington, DC: APA; 2013.
8. Davis RL, Zhong Y. The biology of forgetting—a perspective. Neuron. 2017;95(3):490–503.
9. Higbee KL. Your memory: how it works and how to improve it, 2nd ed. Da Capo Lifelong Books; 2001. p. 33–4.
10. https://icd.who.int/browse11/l-m/en
11. Judge D, Roberts J, Khandker R, et al. Physician perceptions about the barriers to prompt diagnosis of mild cognitive impairment and Alzheimer's disease. Int J AD. 2019;2019:3637954. https://doi.org/10.1155/2019/3637954.
12. https://www.alz.co.uk/adi/pdf/Dementia-Asia-Pacific-2014.pdf
13. https://www.nia.nih.gov/health/what-happens-brain-alzheimers-disease

Chapter 2
Dementia Due to Alzheimer's Disease (AD)

2.1 Presentation and Progression of AD

An accurate and timely diagnosis is a prerequisite for good dementia care. Many people with dementia are never diagnosed. Many receive a diagnosis when it is too late for them to make decisions about their future or to benefit from interventions. Timely diagnosis allows people benefit from treatments that can reduce or delay the progression of cognitive and neuropsychiatric symptoms and avert crises. Additionally, knowing their diagnosis helps families to understand their relatives' behaviour and allow them to access therapies and improve their coping skills.

Barriers and benefits of early diagnosis are summarised in Box 2.1.

Box 2.1 Barriers and Benefits of Timely Dementia Diagnosis
Benefits (*Source: Alzheimer's World Report* [1], *2011*)
- *Optimising current medical management*
- *Relief gained from better understanding of symptoms*
- *Maximising decision-making autonomy*
- *Access to services*
- *Risk reduction*
- *Planning for the future*
- *Improving clinical outcomes*
- *Avoiding or reducing future costs*
- *Diagnosis is a human right*

A. Jha, K. Mukhopadhaya, *Alzheimer's Disease*,
https://doi.org/10.1007/978-3-030-56739-2_2

Barriers
- *No access to medical care*
- *People believe the symptoms are an inevitable part of ageing*
- *Denial of problems*
- *Reluctance to see a doctor due to fear of the diagnosis and concerns about stigma*

2.2 Role of Frontline/Non-specialist Physicians

There is an important question whether frontline physicians in non-specialist settings should make the diagnosis of dementia, in particular early Alzheimer's disease. In low and middle-income countries, it is not possible to have sufficient manpower to run specialist memory services. With a disorder as common as dementia it is logical to assume that frontline physicians should be enabled to assess and diagnose people with suspected Alzheimer's disease. The ground reality, however, is that primary care physicians, even in high-income countries are reluctant to be directly involved in the diagnosis and treatment of dementia for the following reasons:

- *The belief that nothing can be done for dementia;*
- *Risk avoidance;*
- *Concerns about competency; and*
- *Concerns about the availability of resources*

2.2.1 Presentation of Alzheimer's Disease

Dementia due to Alzheimer's disease is the commonest of the early-onset (before age 65 years) as well as late-onset primary dementias. Given the exponential increase in incidence after age 75, the vast majority of people with AD are elderly. At all ages, females outnumber males by a ratio of 3:1. For all types, the onset is usually insidious and can be dated only imprecisely. The slow development of the intellectual deterioration often allows the patient to preserve considerable social competence until the disease is well advanced. Three main phases of the disease are commonly distinguished—early stage (lasting 2–3 years), middle, and terminal stage in which the patient becomes bedridden and doubly incontinent. In early stages, *failing memory and lack of initiative and interest* are regarded by patients and families as accentuation of the normal processes of ageing.

Preclinical Alzheimer's disease occurs when there are early Alzheimer's pathogenic changes in the brain but no clinical manifestations. These pathogenic changes include extracellular deposition of amyloid β($A\beta$ protein) from cleaved amyloid precursor protein, which is the main component of plaques, and intracellular accumulation of tau protein, which is the main constituent of tangles. These abnormal proteins are being used as diagnostic *biomarkers* (Box 2.2).

Box 2.2 AD Biomarkers

The 'classic' biomarker in medicine is a laboratory parameter that we use for diagnostic purposes. For example, the detection of 'rheumatoid factors' has been an important diagnostic marker for rheumatoid arthritis. Like rheumatoid arthritis, Alzheimer's disease begins with an early, symptom-free phase. In such chronic diseases, biomarkers help to identify high-risk individuals reliably and timely so that they can be treated as soon as possible. There are different types of biomarkers—imaging biomarkers (CT, MRI, PET) or molecular biomarkers with three subtypes, volatile (like breath), body fluid (like CSF) and biopsy biomarkers. Currently, we have biomarkers for amyloid pathology—Aβ PET and CSF Aβ42/Aβ40. However, CSF and PET examinations are far from routine use. Therefore, blood-based biomarkers are being explored.

Alzheimer's disease has an insidious onset and most people pass through a preclinical asymptomatic phase when cerebral Aβ42 and other abnormal proteins are accumulating in the brain, followed by mild cognitive impairment, and ultimately progress to dementia. Abnormal biomarkers are common, with 10–30% of cognitively healthy people, having substantial brain amyloid deposits on PET scanning. However, most PET- positive people do not decline clinically over the following 18–36 months.

2.2.2   Presenting Symptoms of AD

As a general physician, when you first see a patient in the clinic, you may not have any information apart from their age and gender. You may not even know whether the patient wanted to see you or has been coerced by the family. The presentations may range from fever to forgetfulness or palpitation to psychosis. This, for instance, may be the first and foremost difference between specialist and non-specialist settings—between a general medical clinic in the Indian subcontinent and the specialist memory clinic in the UK. On top of that, you have only about 20 min for the initial assessment while we have at least an hour or so for every new patient.

2.2.2.1   Clinical Presentation

People with dementia may experience memory problems themselves and self-refer to your clinic or their family members may become concerned and suggest that they have an assessment. Some patients may become acutely ill with delirium, which may complicate an underlying dementing illness. The primary care response to presenting problems is shaped by the patient's response to their illness as well as their family member's concerns and expectations. A style of assessment should be adopted that the patient is most comfortable with. There may be a range of barriers preventing the patient accepting the initial assessment, particularly where denial or lack of insight is present. Difficulties can also arise when the presenting symptoms are disruptive of relationships or include paranoia or anxiety.

The commonest clinical presentation of dementia due to Alzheimer's disease is with impairment of memory or more general disorganisation of intellect. Memory problems are usually noted first by relatives than the patient themselves. Examples include missed appointments, unawareness of recent events, tendency to mix up times or to lose or misplace things. More general cognitive decline manifest as loss of overall efficiency, failure to speak coherently or to fail to grasp essentials. Sometimes, relatives notice subtle changes in personality as deterioration in manners or diminished awareness of the needs and feelings of others. Typical early signs are loss of interest and initiative, or inability to perform up to the usual standard, or minor episodes of muddle and confusion (Box 2.3: *Case 1*). Occasionally, the earliest change is noted as the exaggeration of long-standing personality traits such as suspiciousness or egocentricity.

Box 2.3 Case 1: Changes in Memory and Personal Care [2]

A daughter Sarla lives in the USA with her husband. She shares her story about her mother in-law's Alzheimer's disease progressed [2].

"In September 2005, when I visited my in-laws in Delhi, I found 'Amma' to be a little quieter. She showed some signs of memory loss. But Papa insisted she was mostly OK, and this was just ageing. He was a tough person and wanted to appear even tougher to his children who lived far away so they did not worry. My husband visited in December 2005, and they celebrated the parents' wedding anniversary. Amma displayed most of her spirit and dry wit. In spite of the fun they were having, my husband felt that Papa was trying to tell him something but could not draw it out of him. When my husband returned to the USA, he told me, "I guess Amma is having some memory loss, but they are hanging in there".

The turning point came in May 2006, when Didi (elder sister) went to an extended family function and saw Amma dressed in a non-matching salwar kameez. This made her take notice as Amma was 'looking bad' in front of so many other relatives. In the last few months, Amma had been unable to take a bath herself. She had no awareness of personal hygiene and would go out with uncombed hair.

Papa finally told us that she would wake up in the middle of the night and get violent with him. All these symptoms were disturbing and completely new to us—we did not know what was happening".

2.2.3 Five A's of Alzheimer's

A typical presentation of Alzheimer's disease consists of an *'early significant and progressive **episodic memory deficit** (to be discussed later) that remains dominant in the later stages of the disease and is followed by or associated with other cognitive impairments*. They are often considered as the five As of Alzheimer's: ***amnesia, aphasia, apraxia, agnosia*** **and** ***abnormal executive function*** (Fig. 2.1). Clinical assessment of these signs will be discussed in the assessment chapter.

2.2.3.1 Amnesia

Memory impairment (Amnesia), especially for recent events, with relative sparing of working memory, is an invariable and early symptom of AD. The primary neuropsychological deficit is one of encoding and storing memories rather than failure to retrieve. As the disease progresses, even more remote memories are lost and amnesia manifests as *episodic, semantic* and *visuospatial deficits*. Episodic memory is the memory of events and there is a gradient for loss, with more recent events being lost before more remote events.

The emphasis on episodic memory deficits as a core feature arises from empirical evidence that the medial temporal lobes are typically the first structure affected by AD pathology before it cascades to other cortical areas.

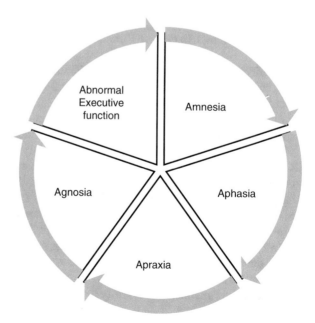

Fig. 2.1 Five A's of Alzheimer's

2.2.3.2   Aphasia

The earliest changes are word finding difficulties and at this stage syntax may appear superficially intact, but close analyses may reveal unfinished sentences, inappropriate usage of tense and other minor errors. As the disease progresses, *receptive* difficulties become increasingly apparent and in the final stages of the disease, speech becomes increasingly impaired with *perseverations, echolalia, decreased fluency and non-speech verbalisations.*

2.2.3.3   Apraxia

Difficulties with complex motor tasks not due to primary motor deficits resulting in increasingly poor self-care and risk of harm. In the early stages this may be elicited by asking the patient to enact a command (*ideomotor apraxia*).

2.2.3.4   Agnosia

The failure to correctly interpret a sensory input, or *agnosia*, is common in AD, especially *prosopagnosia* (failure to recognise familiar faces). When patients misinterpret their reflection in the mirror as a stranger, it is known as '*mirror sign,*' caused by *autoprosopagnosi*a, failure to recognise one's own face.

2.2.3.5   Abnormal Executive Function

The ability to plan, to organise and to maintain attention are lost early and consistently in AD. Executive functioning is a frontal lobe function. A predominance of executive dysfunction and aphasia with relative sparing of memory suggests a *frontal lobe predominant dementia*. Frontal lobe function can be tested by asking the patient to copy hand sequences (as discussed later under RUDAS).

Whatever the form of presentation, dementia may appear abruptly even though its evolution has been insidious. Relatives may have adjusted to the slow decline until some sort of crisis forces them to realise the truth. As the disorder progresses, changes in emotional control and social awareness are also noted. There may also be impaired capacity for decision making, concentration and comprehension. Thinking becomes slow with ready mental fatigue. The content of thought becomes impoverished with inability to produce new ideas, and a tendency to follow set topics and memories from the past. The ability to argue and reason logically is impaired. Likewise, the ability to keep in mind various aspects of a situation simultaneously is also affected. Intellectual flexibility is lost, leading to difficulty in shifting from one frame of reference to another. Abstract ideas present especial difficulty and concepts tend to be given their most literal interpretation. Judgement is impaired and the patient may not be aware of their illness at all. Anxiety, depression and agitation also become common. Irritability leads to outbursts of anger and hostility (Box 2.4: Case 2).

Box 2.4 Case 2: Strange Behaviour [2]

Rajesh is a management consultant living in Bangalore. His mother-in-law started showing dementia symptoms about 13 years ago and was diagnosed 10 years ago. Rajesh shares how he failed to support his wife in the beginning.

"My mother-in-law suffers from dementia, and my wife is the primary care-giver. After she was diagnosed, and my wife took over the role of the primary caregiver, I failed to support her for many years because of ignorance and some incorrect attitude. My ignorance affected many of my actions and decisions.

- *When my mother in-law's behaviour became stranger and embarrassing, I thought of her as "difficult person to live with". It was only after she started confusing morning and evening and could no longer read the time on a clock that I acknowledged her medical condition. But even then, I did not think her agitation, frustration and "lies" were actually the impact of dementia.*
- *I did not realize that dementia gets worse with time. So I did not plan for the fact that her care would also keep increasing.*
- *My ignorance also meant that I could no longer talk with my mother-in-law. I began avoiding her because of her "unreasonable" behaviour. It was many years before I figured out how to communicate with her."*

Emotional lability may be extreme with episodes of abnormal laughing and crying for little or no cause. The "*catastrophic reaction*" may be observed when the patient is unable to cope with the situation. He may over-react in an anxious aggressive manner, or alternatively become quiet and withdrawn.

In the later stages hygiene and personal appearance are neglected leading to urinary and faecal incontinence. Thinking becomes incoherent and disorganised. Eventually, behaviour becomes futile and aimless often with mannerisms and stereotypies.

Central to the diagnosis of a dementing disorder in the elderly patient is determining the presence of disorders in memory and other cognitive processes, such as language, visuospatial perception, and personality. The task of detecting symptoms is simplified to some extent in the advanced stages of dementia; diagnosing dementia is much more challenging for the clinician when the symptoms are far less obvious. Equally challenging is the clinical distinction between different subtypes of dementia that present in similar manners, such as frontotemporal dementia for which no drug treatment is currently available.

Because of its slow and insidious onset, the early stages of Alzheimer's disease can be confused with relatively benign memory impairments that are associated with normal ageing. The early symptomatic phase of Alzheimer's disease, commonly referred as mild cognitive impairment, can be indistinguishable on bedside clinical examination from normal ageing, but the disease is more readily identified by means of neuropsychological testing with or without the aid of other diagnostic procedures, such as CT, MRI or PET scans.

As you can see, a clinician needs both clinical skills and basic understanding of the neuroscience for an effective dementia assessment. Cognitive testing is useful not only to assist in diagnosing dementia, but also as an objective baseline for tracking changes over a period of time. Finally, cognitive test is also helpful in monitoring treatment response.

2.3 Natural History/Progression of AD

Time from diagnosis to death varies from studies to studies. In tertiary clinical centres, it is on the order of 10–12 years, while it varies from only *3–5 years* in population studies, because significant proportion of patients with AD do not make it to clinical centres. A significant number of patients exhibit slow progression after the onset of dementia. In a Canadian study [3], 25–30% of individuals exhibited limited to no progression from milder stages of dementia even 3–5 years after onset.

A significant number of patients exhibit slow progression after the onset of dementia. Dementia affects each person in a different way, depending upon the impact of the disease and the person's premorbid health and personality. The problems linked to dementia can be understood in three stages (Fig. 2.2): *early, middle and late* (WHO dementia Report [4], 2012, p. 7).

2.3.1 Early Stage of Dementia

The early stage is often overlooked. Relatives and friends (as well as professionals) see it as "old age", just a normal part of ageing process. People in early stage of dementia:

- Become forgetful, especially regarding things that just happened
- May have some difficulty with communication, such as difficulty in finding words
- Become lost in familiar places
- Lose track of the time, including time of the day, month, year, season
- Have difficulty making decisions and handling personal finances
- Have difficulty carrying out complex household tasks
- Mood and behaviour changes: may become less active and motivated and lose interest in activities and hobbies; may show mood changes, including depression and anxiety; may react unusually angrily or aggressively on occasion

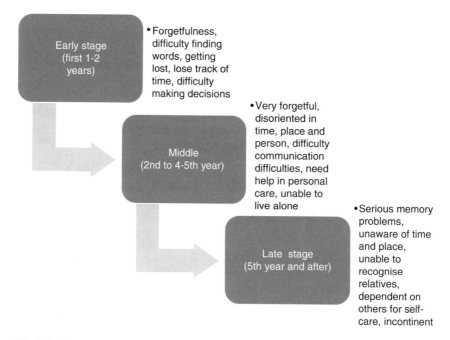

Fig. 2.2 Common symptoms reported in different stages of dementia (WHO, 2012 [4])

2.3.2 Middle Stage of Dementia

As the disease progresses, limitations become clearer and more restricting. People:

- Become very forgetful, especially of recent events and people's names
- Have difficulty comprehending time, date, place and events; may become lost at home as well as in the community
- Have increasing difficulty with communication (speech and comprehension)
- Need help with personal care (i.e. toileting, washing, dressing)
- Unable to successfully prepare food, cook, clean or shop
- Unable to live alone safely without considerable support
- Behaviour changes may include wandering, repeated questioning, calling out, clinging, disturbed sleeping, hallucinations
- May display inappropriate behaviour in the home or in the community (e.g. disinhibition, aggression)

2.3.3 Late Stage of Dementia

The last stage is of nearly total dependence and inactivity. Memory disturbances are very serious, and the physical side of the disease becomes more obvious. People are:

- Usually unaware of time and lace
- Have difficulty understanding what is happening around them
- Unable to recognise relatives, friends and familiar objects
- Unable to eat without assistance, may have difficulty swallowing
- Increasing need for assisted self-care (bathing and toileting)
- May have bladder and bowel incontinence
- Change in mobility, may be unable to walk or be confined to a wheelchair or bed
- Behaviour changes, may escalate and include aggression towards carer, nonverbal agitation (kicking, hitting, screaming or moaning)
- Unable to find his or her way around the home

These periods are given as an approximate guideline only—sometimes people may deteriorate more quickly, sometimes more slowly. Also, not all persons with dementia will display all the symptoms.

References

1. https://www.alz.co.uk/research/world-report-2011
2. www.dementiacarenotes.in
3. Tschanz JT, Corcoran CD, Schwartz S, et al. Progression of cognitive, functional, and neuropsychiatric symptom domains in a population cohort with Alzheimer's dementia: the cache county dementia progression study. Am J Geriatr Psychiatry. 2011;19(6):532–42.
4. https://www.who.int/mental_health/publications/dementia_report_2012/en/

Chapter 3
Dementia Assessment

3.1 Assessment: The OBAMA Index

Assessment is not a mysterious process—it is quite mundane and just needs to be done properly. It is helpful for the clinician to be familiar with couple of cognitive tools since it is unrealistic to do anything but a brief 'screen' in a normal primary care consultation. Being able to draw a perfect clock, to all intents and purposes, renders a diagnosis of dementia unlikely. Drug therapy, particularly with memory drugs, is straightforward and well within the capabilities of general practitioners.
      Dr Elizabeth Barrett & Professor Burns, Dementia Revealed [1]

Assessing a person with suspected dementia may be daunting for the uninitiated as it puts you in an unfamiliar territory. This is where you need to recall all clinical assessment skills, including neurological and psychiatric skills. You will have to work as three in one—a physician, a neurologist and a psychiatrist—all at once. But it is not mysterious. You need to have a high index of suspicion of possible dementia and a structure in your head to assess the person's cognition. Whenever you see an elderly patient (especially aged 75 and over), in your clinic for any health problem, please think of dementia by remembering the mnemonic **OBAMA**, which stands for:

- **O**ld age
- **B**ehaviour change
- **A**bsent mindedness (minor forgetfulness)
- **M**emory problems and,
- **Activity** problems (at home and work)

Recently, like MCI, the concept of "Mild Behavioural Impairment (MBI) [2]" has been proposed to describe people at an increased risk of dementia due to the presence of late life acquired neuropsychiatric symptoms, such as **apathy, affective symptoms, impulse control problems,** *or* **social inappropriateness.** *These may be symptoms of prodromal dementia.*

Dementia is a group of neurodegenerative disorders that are characterized by progressive cognitive impairment and loss of ability to perform activities of daily living. The diagnosis of Alzheimer's disease (AD) is a three-stage process. First the general evidence for the dementia syndrome is gathered, then depression and delirium are excluded, and finally the clinical presentation is examined to see if it fits the diagnostic criteria for AD—*insidious onset and gradual progression in the absence of other possible causes.* Such distinctions are important because depression and delirium require immediate attention and other types of dementia have different treatment and prognosis.

Mental, neurological and substance use (MNS) disorders are highly prevalent accounting for a large burden of disease and disability globally. There remains a wide gap between available resources and the large need for services for people with MNS disorders. More than 45% of the world population lives in a country where there is less than one psychiatrist for every 100,000 people and there are even fewer neurologists. It is not possible for specialists alone to provide services for people affected by MNS disorders, especially in low- and middle-income countries (LMICs).

To bridge this gap, the WHO launched the Mental Health Gap Action Programme (mhGAP) in 2008. Subsequently, the *WHO mhGap Intervention Guide* [3] was created as a simple step by step guidance for priority MNS disorders, including dementia. WHO member countries are expected to organise dementia training for their primary health care professionals. If not already done, you may like to request your local psychiatrists or neurologists to provide such training for you. The key principles of dementia care are outlined in as Box 3.1.

Box 3.1 WHO Principles of Dementia Care
- *Early diagnosis* in order *to promote early and optimal management*
- *Optimising health, cognition, activity and wellbeing*
- *Identifying and treating accompanying physical illness*
- *Detecting and treating behavioural and psychological symptoms*
- *Providing information and long-term support to carers*

Early diagnosis of dementia is essential for its optical management. A process of assessment and reassessment is the basis of management since dementia is a progressive condition. In the present chapter we focus on the initial assessment.

Conducting an assessment for dementia involves the following steps. First, a precise description of the presenting problems, their nature, and history of their onset is gathered. This is followed by a history of past MNS issues, general health problems, family MNS history, and psychosocial history. While taking the history from the patient, a general physical and mental state examination can also be done. As part of the dementia assessment, always conduct a physical examination and organise basic laboratory tests as needed. The assessment should be always conducted with informed consent of the person.

> *The clinical interview is the soul of any dementia assessment. The first step is usually to elicit a complete history of signs and symptoms, recalled by the patient and/or an informant. A highly skilled interviewer structures the interaction as a conversation, establishing rapport and confidence.*

In addition to the clinical assessment, a *functional assessment* is also required to establish the patient's strengths and weaknesses. A standardized functional assessment tools, such as FAQ (to be discussed later), help in the diagnosis of dementia. Functional activity reflects motor, perceptual skills, cognitive abilities, and general wellbeing. It has two main aspects: *basic* and *instrumental*. The basic activities of daily living (BADL) comprise of self-care and self-maintenance skills such as washing, bathing, dressing, maintaining continence, eating, transferring, grooming. On the other hand, the more complex skills are required to live independently in the community—the instrumental activities of daily living (IADL). The four domains of IADL significantly associated with cognitive impairment are: *managing medication, using the telephone, coping with budget,* and *using transportation.*

Involvement of patients in information exchange and decision-making at all stages of their illness is good practice and the value of maintaining a truthful relationship with a patient should be part of professional practice. At the outset of assessment, it is helpful to seek permission for disclosure to family or friends.

3.2 Steps of Clinical Assessment

> ***Communication Tips***: *People with dementia have cognitive impairments that limit the communication they can have with you. Therefore, make an effort to communicate with the person **and** their carer. Make sure you sit in a way that the person can see and hear you properly. Speak clearly, slowly and with eye contact. Look at the body language and non-verbal cues. Give the caregiver and family a chance to talk and listen to their concerns. Be flexible in your approach with the carer and family. The family may come to you with needs you did not expect.*

WHO Dementia Guide recommends the following steps:

3.2.1 Step 1: History Taking

(a) Presenting Complaints
Main symptoms or reason that the person/informant is seeking care.
- *Ask when, why, and how it started.*

(*Clinical tip*: it may not be easy for carers to remember the sequence of events around the onset of AD. What happened when, in what order. John Bayley, for instance, writes about his famous actress wife in his book, *IRIS: A Memoir of Iris Murdoch* (1999). *"The condition seems to get into the narrative, producing repetition and preoccupied query"*.)

- *How old was the person when they first noticed the symptoms?*
- *Did the symptom start suddenly or gradually?*
- *How long have the symptoms been present for?*
- *Are the symptoms worse at night?*
- *Is their associated drowsiness, impairment of consciousness?*

Examples
- *"I can't remember a thing; I am afraid of talking to people, in case I will ask the same question again; It's so embarrassing."*

"I know what to say but it does not come out. I get very frustrated and angry because of this"

Clinical tip: At times, people who complain bitterly of poor memory are most likely to suffer from depression, anxiety or hypochondriasis. People with dementia often lack insight and play down cognitive difficulties they are experiencing. An independent informant in this situation is essential. For example, consider the following example:

A patient: *"I don't think that I have any real problem at all with my memory."*
Her husband: *"She has bad short memory and repeats herself all the time. She puts things away and blames others for moving them."*

Similarly, another patient was convinced that she carried out all the domestic chores that she used to do in the past. In reality, her husband did all the cooking, washing, shopping and assisted her to dress and wash. Without his help, she could not cope alone.

Ask the Carer
- Have you noticed a change in person's ability to think and reason?
- Does the person often forget where they have put things?
- Does the person forget what happened the day before?
- Does the person forget where they are?
- Does the person get confused?
- Does the person have difficulty dressing (misplacing buttons, putting clothes on the wrong way)?
- How has the person changed since having these symptoms (changed behaviours, ability to reason, changed personality, changed emotional control)?
- What does the person do in a typical day? How do they behave? Is this different from what they used to do?

(b) **Past MNS History**

- *Ask about similar problems in the past, and psychiatric hospitalisations or medications prescribed for MNS conditions, and any past depressive episodes.*
- *Explore tobacco, alcohol and substance use.*

Recent research [4] suggests that risk factors for progression to dementia depends on gender of the person. Risk of dementia is higher in men with history of stroke and in women with history of depression and previous use of anticholinergic medication.

(c) **General Health History**

- *Ask about physical health problems and medications.*
- *Obtain a list of current medications.*
- *Ask about allergies to medications.*

(d) **Family History of MNS conditions**

- *Explore possible family history of MNS conditions and ask if anyone had similar symptoms or has received treatment for an MNS condition.*

(e) **Psychosocial History**

- *Ask about current stressors, coping methods and social support.*
- *Ask about current socio-occupational functioning (how the person is functioning at home, work and in relationships)*
- *Obtain basic information including where the person lives, level of education, work/employment history, marital status and number/ages of children, income, and household structure/living conditions.*

3.2.2 Step 2: Physical Examination

Persons with MNS disorders are at a higher risk of premature mortality from preventable diseases and therefore must always receive physical health assessment to identify concurrent conditions and educate the person about preventive measures. **Cardiovascular risk factors include hypertension, high cholesterol, diabetes, smoking, obesity, heart disease (chest pain, heart attack, previous stroke or transient ischaemic attack, TIA).** Key points to remember are:

- Ask about risk factors including *physical inactivity, inappropriate diet, tobacco, harmful use of alcohol, and chronic disease.*
- *Perform physical examination.*
- *Consider a differential diagnosis*
- Rule out physical conditions and underlying causes of dementia presentation by history, physical examination and basic laboratory tests as needed and available.
- *Identify comorbidities*

- Often, a person may have more than one MNS condition at the same time. It is important to assess and manage this when it occurs.

  As a minimum the following points should be noted routinely:

- Pulse rate and blood pressure
- Signs of hemiparesis, hemianesthesia or sensory inattention suggest cerebrovascular disease or space occupying lesion
- Increased tones in the limbs is either due to antipsychotic medication or raises the possibility of Lewy body dementia
- Finally, observe the gait:

  - Difficulty rising from a seat without support of arms, hesitation on starting to walk, a shuffling gait and lack of arm swinging are the features of Parkinson's disease, suggest a diagnosis of either dementia in Parkinson's disease or Lewy body dementia.
  - Normal pressure hydrocephalus is characterised by an ataxic and apraxic gait
  - Persistently bumping into objects on one side gives a suspicion of visual defect or neglect

It is important to establish whether the patient has features of hypothyroidism: clinical history of goitre, slow pulse and dry skin.

3.2.3 Step 3: Mental State Examination

A brief mental state examination adapted for non-specialists include:

- Behaviour and appearance = symptoms and signs involving the way a person looks like or acts
- Mood and affect = symptoms and signs involving expression of emotions or feeling states
- Content of thought = symptoms and signs involving subject matter of thoughts including delusions, paranoia, suspiciousness and suicidal ideation.
- Perceptual disturbance = sensory perceptions occurring in the absence of the appropriate (external) stimulus (e.g. auditory or visual hallucinations). The person may or may not have insight into the unreal nature of the perception
- Cognition = symptoms, signs and clinical findings indicative of a disturbance in attention, memory, judgement, reasoning, problem solving, decision making, comprehension and the integration of these functions.

3.2.4 Step 4: Assess for Signs of Dementia

This is the most important step in any dementia assessment. A traditional medical training does not adequately prepare doctors for meaningful cognitive assessment. It takes both time and energy. A brief cognitive test does not usually take more than 10 min to complete. Yet, even psychiatrists in low-resource countries tend to avoid this crucial step in their busy psychiatric clinics. Perhaps, like our memory nurses in the UK, there is a need to develop an additional pool of '*Memory Clinic Assistants*' to assist non-specialist doctors. These 'Assistants' may be able to conduct and provide a 'cognitive test' result, similar to blood and urine tests commonly done in developing countries.

*The **Memory First Aid International** [5] is trying to train science and psychology graduates in South Asian countries with a view to screen and assess older people with suspected dementia. The WHO is also encouraging member countries to train their primary health care staff in dementia and mental health, using mhGAP Dementia Intervention Guide.*

Dementia diagnosis depends on the direct assessment of cognitive functions by testing memory, orientation, and language skills along with a general neurologic examination.

Example: *Are there problems with memory and orientation? (e.g. forgetting what happened the previous day or not knowing where he or she is).*

Common Presentations
People with dementia can present with problems in:

- **Cognitive function:** Confusion, memory, problems planning.
- **Emotional control**: Mood swings, personality changes.
- **Behaviour**: Wandering, aggression.
- **Physical health**: incontinence, weight loss.
- **Difficulty in performing daily activities**: Ability to cook, clean dishes.

Complaints about poor memory are the most common reason for coming to a physician in non-specialist settings and provide a good starting point for the consultation despite not being very specific. In the early stage of dementia, people usually present with the following features:

- *Becoming forgetful, especially of things that have just happened*
- *Some difficulty with communication (e.g. difficulty in finding words)*
- *Becoming lost and confused in familiar places—may lose items by putting them in unusual places and be unable to find them*
- *Losing track of the time, including time of day, month, year*
- *Difficulty in making decisions and handling personal finances*
- *Having difficulty carrying out familiar tasks at home or work—trouble driving or forgetting how to use appliances in the kitchen*
- *Mood and behaviour:*

  - *Less active and motivated, loses interest in activities and hobbies*
  - *May show mood changes, including depression or anxiety*
  - *May react unusually or aggressively on occasion*

Testing Orientation, Memory and Language
Example of questions:

1. Tell them three words (e.g. boat, house, fish) and ask them to repeat after you.
2. Point to their elbow and ask, *"What do we call this?"*
3. Ask the following questions:

   - *What do you do with a hammer?* (Acceptable answer: "Drive a nail into something").

- *Where is the local market/local store?*
- *What day of the week is it?*
- *What is the season?*
- *Please point first to the window and then the door.*

4. Ask, *"Do you remember the three words I told you a few minutes ago?"*

3.2.5 Step 5: Differential Diagnosis—Delirium and Depression

Consider the differential diagnosis and rule out conditions that have similar presenting symptoms. You need to exclude at least two common conditions encountered in older patients—delirium and depression.

The level of *alertness* during assessment is an important clue to the presence of a delirium or the side effects of medication. Delirium may be marked by both restlessness and distractibility, or apathy (the patient may be quiet). The patient may drift off to sleep easily during the consultation. If there is any concern about the level of alertness of the patient, current medication must be reviewed. It may be misleading and futile to perform a detailed cognitive assessment on a patient with diminished alertness. At this stage, history of the onset and progression of the symptoms become very helpful.

Delirium can be missed in older patients. The *hypoactive* form of delirium is characterised by lethargy and psychomotor retardation. These patients may appear somewhat similar to depressed patients but can be distinguished on the basis of history and mental state examination. A previous history of depressive episode and presence of biological features of depression may help distinguish depression from delirium.

Have the symptoms been present and slowly progressing for at least 6 months?

If NO, Ask for any of the following:

- Abrupt onset
- Short duration (days to weeks)
- Disturbance at night and associated with impairment of consciousness
- Disorientation of time and place

Clinical Tip 1: *Delirium*
Delirium is a transient fluctuating mental state characterised by disturbed attention that develops over a short period of time and tends to fluctuate during the course of a day. It may result from acute organic causes such as infections, medication, metabolic abnormalities, substance intoxication, or substance withdrawal.

Clinical Tip 2: *Depression*
Depression: cognitive impairment may be the result of depression or dementia may present with anxiety and depression. Depressive illness can impair memory, executive function, and cause word finding difficulties. The emergence of mood disorder in later life indicates neurodegenerative disease, particularly Alzheimer's and Parkinson's disease dementia.

Common Presentations of Depression
- *Multiple persistent physical symptoms with no clear cause*
- *Low energy, fatigue, sleep problems*
- *Persistent sadness or low depressed mood, anxiety*
- *Loss of interest or pleasure in activities that are normally pleasurable*

Has the person had several of the following additional symptoms for at least 2 weeks?
- **Disturbed sleep or sleeping too much**
- **Significant change in appetite or weight (decrease or increase)**
- **Beliefs of worthlessness or excessive guilt**
- **Fatigue or loss of energy**
- **Reduced concentration**
- **Indecisiveness**
- **Observable agitation or physical restlessness**
- **Talking or moving more slowly than usual**
- **Hopelessness**
- **Suicidal thoughts or acts**

A person with depression may have psychotic symptoms such as delusions or hallucinations. If present, treatment of depression needs to be adapted.

If those symptoms are present, consider a diagnosis of depression and treat with an appropriate antidepressant.

3.2.6 Basic Laboratory Tests

Request laboratory tests when indicated and possible, especially to rule out physical causes.

If you suspect delirium, evaluate for possible medical causes (toxic/metabolic/ infectious).

- *Obtain urinalysis to evaluate for infection*
- *Review medications, particularly those with significant anticholinergic side effects (such as antidepressants, antihistamines, and antipsychotics)*
- *Evaluate for pain*
- *Evaluate nutritional status, consider vitamin deficiency or electrolyte abnormality*

3.2.6.1   Current Medication

It is vital to check the currently prescribed and non-prescribed treatments by asking both patients and reliable informants to produce their actual medication. It also helps to identify problems with compliance. The use of ayurvedic and homeopathic medicine is not uncommon in the Indian subcontinent. Polite questioning about why these treatments are being taken can give useful insights into current concerns and may raise issues not identified elsewhere. Checking the treatment actually being taken may also reveal an important recent change of medication. The *anticholinergic burden* of commonly prescribed medicines may be calculated using the free *Anticholinergic Effect on Cognition Tool* [6] available at https://medichec.com (Box).

Box Anticholinergic Effect on Cognition (Medichec-AEC) Tool

A number of validated anticholinergic scales exist in order to classify drugs according to their anticholinergic risk. These are generally based on the subjective experience of assessors and are usually dependent on the drug's general potency to muscarinic receptors. Based on a classification developed by Bishara et al. [6], a novel *anticholinergic effect on cognition* (AEC) tool has recently been introduced to identify specifically the anticholinergic effect on cognition for medicines commonly used in the elderly.

The AEC tool classifies medication according to a traffic system, giving drugs an individual score of 0, 1, 2 or 3. A score of 0 means the medication has no anticholinergic effect on cognition, and a score of 3 means it has the most effect. The individual scores of all the medications that a patient is taking are then added together to give a total AEC score of 2 or more, or have a total AEC score of 3 or more, have a medication review so that the offending drugs can be withdrawn or switched to a safer alternative. The aim is to reduce the total AEC score to the lowest possible value.

Bishara and colleagues conducted a quality improvement exercise at a large teaching hospital in London where the introduction of the AEC tool led to an increase in the identification of anticholinergic medication from 11 to 85%. The success of this project led to the development of *Medichec*, a web-based and application version of the ACE tool. This allows clinicians to easily check their patient's medication, and the cumulative anticholinergic burden score is automatically calculated. Currently, Medichec contains over 2000 medications by their generic names listed in the British National Formulary. The AEC tool is available online as a free resource at https://medichec.com. An android and apple versions are supposed to be available.

The abuse of alcohol and benzodiazepines can be a major problem in older patients presenting with cognitive impairment. This should be assessed carefully if the patient lives in an urban area and drives a car. If the patient is driving, it is important to ask others about any concerns they may have or incidents which have occurred and will need to consider whether to ask the patient to stop driving if there are safety concerns.

3.2.7 Genetic Testing

Genetic testing is not recommended in late onset-dementia, because of uncertain benefits and potential harm. The ApoEe4allele is the only genetic factor that increases the susceptibility to late-onset Alzheimer's disease. Testing of patients even with young-onset dementia and unaffected at-risk relatives for genetic causes of dementia is not routinely done.

3.3   Cognitive Screening Instruments

Despite the advances in neuroimaging and biomarkers, a diagnosis of AD continues to rest heavily on cognitive assessment. At present, the most used cognitive screening instrument for the detection of AD is the Mini-Mental State Examination (MMSE). However, MMSE has a very limited ability to differentiate between mild cognitive impairment (MCI) and healthy controls. There is no perfect screening instrument that can be used in every population and for all types of neurodegenerative and cerebrovascular brain diseases.

Clinicians in a non-specialist setting would prefer a quick and easy-to-interpret cognitive test, such as RUDAS (to be described later), whereas in the UK memory clinics we prefer a longer ACE-III which takes up to 30 min. Our advice to non-specialist doctors is to perform a cognitive assessment in two steps—use a screener first, and then a standard test later for screen-positive cases at a separate and longer consultation.

3.3.1 Mini-Cog

For the purpose of this book, we have chosen the *Mini-Cog* [7] (Box 3.2), which is a short (3-min) screening instrument for cognitive impairment in older adults. It consists of two components, a *3-item recall* test for memory and a simply scored *clock drawing test*.

> **Box 3.2 Mini-Cog**
> The Mini-Cog is administered as follows:
>
> 1. *Instruct the patient to listen carefully to and remember three unrelated words (e.g. ball, car, man) and then repeat the words.*
> 2. *Ask the patient to draw the face of a clock, either on a blank sheet of paper or on a sheet with the clock circle already drawn on the page. After the patient puts the numbers on the clock face, ask him/her to draw the hands of the clock to read a specific time (ten past ten is popular as it resembles a smiley face).*
> 3. *Ask the patient to repeat the three previously stated words*
>
> *If the three words are correctly recalled, then this suggests there is no significant cognitive impairment.*
> *If none are recalled, this suggests there is significant impairment.*
> *If 1 or 2 are recalled, use the clock drawing test as an arbiter—if it is normal, then there is unlikely to be significant impairment, if it is abnormal, then further enquiry is needed.*

The test has minimal language content, which reduces cultural and educational bias. It has been translated into several languages and can be used effectively after brief training. We strongly recommend watching a training video, such as the at the YouTube by ACTOnALZ.

3.3.2 RUDAS

The *Rowland Universal Dementia Assessment Scale* [8] (RUDAS, Box 3.3) is a useful instrument particularly for people in low and middle-income countries where literacy or education is low. Its administration and scoring are described in the next section.

> **Box 3.3 RUDAS**
> *Although many instruments are available, most are influenced by age, education, ethnicity and language of interview. Many older people from culturally and linguistically diverse countries have low levels of education and speak little English, and therefore decisions based on these instruments may be misleading. Although, an Indian screening tool—the Dementia Assessment by Rapid Test (DART [9])—has been developed for illiterate population, it has a low specificity at 60% compared to 76% of our preferred tool, RUDAS (Appendix A), described later.*

Table 3.1 Functional activity questionnaire

1. Writing checks, paying bills, balancing check book	
2. Assembling tax records, business affairs, or papers	
3. Shopping alone for clothes, household necessities, or groceries	
4. Playing game of skill, working on a hobby	
5. Heating water, making cup of coffee, turning off stove after use	
6. Preparing balance meal	
7. Keeping track of current events	
8. Paying attention to, understanding, discussing TV, book, magazine	
9. Remembering appointments, family occasions, holidays, medicines	
10. Travelling out of neighbourhood, driving, arranging to take buses	
Total score	

3.3.3 Functional Assessment: FAQ

Valid and reliable clinical information about functional ability is essential for a diagnosis of dementia. One of the defining features of mild cognitive impairment (MCI) that distinguishes it from mild dementia is the requirement for 'essentially intact' activities of daily living (ADL). Basic ADL consists of activities such as dressing, grooming, bathing, toileting, and feeding oneself, while instrumental activities of daily living (IADLs), consists of activities such as preparing meals, performing household chores, running errands, travelling outside of one's neighbourhood, keeping track of one's schedule and appointments, managing finances, and doing the taxes. Many IADLs scales have been validated for the assessment of functional impairment in dementia. NICE recommends that when taking history from someone who knows the person with suspected dementia, consider supplementing this with a structured instrument such as the *Functional Activities Questionnaire* [10] (**FAQ**).

Functional changes that require a higher cognitive ability compared to basic activities of daily living, are noted earlier in the dementia process with IADLs. This tool is useful to monitor these functional changes over time. The IADLs are better preserved in MCI than in mild AD, but the precise threshold of functional decline that separates MCI from dementia is difficult to determine without objective structured assessment. The FAQ may be used to differentiate those with mild cognitive impairment and mild Alzheimer's disease. The FAQ is a consistently accurate instrument with good sensitivity (85%) and high reliability (exceeding 0.90). However, as with other instruments that measure functional activities using indirect approaches, there may be over or under estimation of abilities because of the lack of direct observations. Table 3.1 provides the details of the FAQ:

3.3.4 Functional Activities Questionnaire [10]

3.3.4.1 Administration

Ask informant to rate patient's ability using the following scoring system:

- Dependent = 3
- Requires assistance = 2
- Has difficulty but does by self = 1
- Normal = 0
- Never did [the activity] but could do now = 0
- Never did and would have difficulty now = 1

Evaluation
Sum scores (range 0–30). Cut off point of **9** (dependent in 3 or more activities) is recommended to indicate impaired function and possible cognitive impairment.

3.3.5 ECG

An ECG is mainly useful in assessing heart rhythm and rate prior to prescribing medication for AD, especially an Acetylcholinesterase inhibitor (AChEI). ECG is helpful because AChEIs tend to slow the heat rate and may cause syncope. Box 3.4 provides the practical advice to GPs given by the NHS England.

Box 3.4 NHS England's Advice [11] on ECG
- *Acetylcholinesterase inhibitors should be used with great caution if the pulse rate is <60 bpm.*
- *If the pulse rate is >70 bpm and regular there is no necessity to undertake an ECG.*
- *If the pulse rate is <70 bpm, or irregular, an ECG is required.*
- *If there is a conduction abnormality, or an abnormal rhythm, specialist advice should be sought.*
- *It is usually safe to prescribe when atrial fibrillation is well controlled, providing the pulse is above 60.*
- *If the patient is on beta-blockers it may be worthwhile considering a reduction in dose to keep the pulse rate >60.*

Ischaemic changes and atrial fibrillation need to be noted. Left bundle branch block indicates ischaemic damage and risk. For the purposes of a non-specialist setting, first or second-degree heart block, or a heart rate of less than **60/min** should be considered *contraindications* to treatment with AChEIs.

3.3.6 Neuroimaging (CT and MRI Scans)

Most national guidelines suggest that structural neuroimaging is part of routine clinical assessment, although in many areas access to neuroimaging is not feasible. Some countries—e.g. Canada—do not recommend the routine use of neuroimaging.

CT scans are cheaper, quicker (helpful if patients have trouble lying flat or remaining still) and can be used in those with pacemakers. However, *MRI is the preferred imaging method for early diagnosis* because of its greater sensitivity and ability to differentiate dementia subtypes, especially for those with vascular lesions.

The pattern of regional brain atrophy helps to distinguish the common neurodegenerative causes of dementia. Disproportional hippocampal atrophy suggests AD rather than vascular dementia or dementia with Lewy bodies, but there is overlap. Rates of brain atrophy on serial MRI are increased (3–4 times) in AD relative to normal ageing. A repeat scan after a year might clarify the diagnosis, especially the conversion from MCI to AD. Medial temporal lobe atrophy on MRI also differentiates Alzheimer's disease from healthy ageing.

3.3.7 Functional and Molecular Imaging

Positron Emission Tomography imaging (PET) has recently been incorporated into dementia workup, and imaging agents that specifically bind amyloid or tau are being studied to determine their clinical utility. The main risk of PET imaging is exposure from radioactive imaging agents, such as flurodeoxyglucose used as a radiotracer (*FDG-PET*), which has a half-life of about 110 min. It permits in-vivo assessment of brain metabolism and supports assessment of frontotemporal dementia, particularly when clinical assessment is uncertain and there is little change on structural imaging. It shows focal frontal or temporal hypometabolism, or both. FDG-PET was approved by the UK NICE guideline in 2018.

Functional imaging is helpful clinically in distinguishing dementia with Lewy bodies from other causes of dementia because dopamine depletion can be detected by dopamine transporter (*DAT*) scans. In moderate dementia, when dementia with Lewy bodies is suspected, a normal DAT scan reliably excludes dementia with Lewy bodies.

3.4 Assessment Summary

Diagnosis of Alzheimer's dementia requires structured history taking, mental state examination, physical examination (including neurological), cognitive tests, and blood screening. Results of cognitive testing should be interpreted in the light of premorbid education, language, and literary skills, and any current motor, hearing, and visual impairment. If unsure about the diagnosis, consider referring the patient to the nearest specialist for CT head scan. Vascular changes often coexist with Alzheimer's disease, but a diagnosis of vascular dementia *requires demonstration of major infarcts, a substantial burden (>25%) of white matter lesions, or many lacunae or strategic infarcts.*

In some patients it is not possible to reach a firm diagnosis after a single cognitive assessment, even in specialist memory clinics. This is particularly true for the mild stages of Alzheimer's disease, and reflects the relative insensitivity of both clinical and imaging assessment to early pathology. The time-honoured method of longitudinal follow up and repeated assessment in such cases is invaluable and should not be disregarded.

References

1. https://www.england.nhs.uk/wp-content/uploads/2014/09/dementia-revealed-toolkit.pdf
2. Ismail Z, Smith EE, Geda Y, et al.; The ISTAART Neuropsychiatric Symptoms Professional Interest Area. Neuropsychiatric symptoms as early manifestations of emergent dementia: provisional diagnostic criteria for mild behavioural impairment. Alzheimers Dement. 2016;12:195–202.
3. https://www.who.int/publications/i/item/mhgap-intervention-guide%2D%2D-version-2.0
4. Artero S, Ancelin ML, Portet F, et al. Risk profiles for mild cognitive impairment and progression to dementia are gender specific. J Neurol Neurosurg Psychiatry. 2008;79:979–84.
5. https://www.memoryfirstaid.uk
6. Bishara D, Scott C, Stewart R, et al. Safe prescribing in cognitively vulnerable patients: the use of the anticholinergic effect on cognition (AEC) tool in older adult mental health services. BJPsych Bulletin. 2020;44:26–30.
7. https://mini-cog.com
8. Komalasari R, et al. A review of the Rowland Universal Dementia Assessment Scale. Dementia. 2019;18(7–8):3143–58.
9. Swati B, Sreenivas V, Manjari T, Ashima N. Dementia Assessment by Rapid Test (DART): an Indian screening tool for dementia. J Alzheimers Dis Parkinsonism. 2015;5:198.
10. Pfeffer RI, et al. Measurement of functional activities in older adults in the community. J Gerontol. 1982;37(3):323–9.
11. https://www.england.nhs.uk/wp-content/uploads/2015/01/dementia-diag-mng-ab-pt.pdf

Chapter 4
RUDAS Cognitive Scale

4.1 RUDAS: Rowland Universal Dementia Assessment Scale (Appendix A)

For non-specialist settings, especially in Nepal and India, we recommend the use RUDAS.

> *Ideally, one should learn the cognitive assessment skill by directly observing an experienced clinician and practicing it under supervision.*

You may like to watch the training video RUDAS produced by the South Western Sydney Local Health District. You can get a range of other information at www.rudas.com.au. RUDAS can be translated into any local language without following back-translating procedure.

RUDAS is a six-item (totalling 30 points), interview-based short cognitive instrument. It is designed to minimise the effects of cultural learning and language diversity on the assessment of baseline cognitive performance. RUDAS includes items that address several cognitive domains, including *memory, language, visuospatial orientation, praxis, visuospatial drawing,* and *judgement.* Moreover, all items can be *directly translated* to other languages, without the need to change the structure or the format of any item. It also provides an objective measure of cognitive results that does not rely on history from an informant. *RUDAS is easy to administer, takes around 10 min to administer, and requires minimal training to administer.* A cut off point of **22 or less** indicates cognitive impairment.

RUDAS has been translated in Nepalese language [1] and a cross-culturally adapted Nepali version (N-RUDAS) is available. The original 'cube drawing' test has been replaced with more acceptable 'stick design test' and has an internal consistency of 0.7.

A. Jha, K. Mukhopadhaya, *Alzheimer's Disease*, https://doi.org/10.1007/978-3-030-56739-2_4

4.1.1 Administration and Interpretation of RUDAS

When administering RUDAS it is important to encourage patients to communicate in the language in which they are most competent and comfortable. If, as the test administrator, you are multilingual, you will need to be careful when translating the RUDAS questions as you might find it more difficult when you to read in one language and speak in another. It is important that you *translate* the RUDAS questions precisely.

This section will introduce some of the key components of cognitive impairment characteristic of Alzheimer's dementia.

4.1.1.1 Item 1: Memory

Complaints about memory decline are the most frequent reason for patients coming to a memory clinic. It provides a good starting point despite not being very specific. The ability to register, retain and retrieve information is assessed by two simple tests: *memory registration* and *memory recall*. The patient's capacity for current memorising (new learning) has the most important clinical implications and warrants close attention. Repeat the test item when the first five responses are unsatisfactory.

It is important to ask structured questions as provided in RUDAS.

RUDAS Item 1: Memory Registration
1. (Instructions) *I want you to imagine that we are going shopping. Here is a list of grocery items. I would like you to remember the following items which we need to get from the shop. When we get to the shop in about 5 min-time I will ask you what it is that we have to buy. You must remember the list for me.*
   Tea, Cooking oil, Egg, Soap
   Please repeat this list for me (ask the person to repeat the list three times).
(If the person did not repeat all four words, repeat the list until the person has learned them and can repeat them, or, up to a maximum of five times.)

This is the learning part of the memory question (immediate memory). It is important to give enough learning trials so that the patient registers and retains the list as well as they can (maximum of 5 learning trials).

Poor registration, usually a feature of poor attention or executive dysfunction, may invalidate the results of recall or recognition which test episodic memory. Free recall is harder than the recognition of an item from a list. Testing in the deaf person is not easy, but verbal testing by the use of written instructions, in large print, can be used if the patient is *literate.*

> **Working Memory**
> Lapses in concentration and attention (losing one's train of thought, wandering into a room and forgetting the reason, forgetting a phone number which has just been looked at) are common and increase with age, depression, and anxiety. Such symptoms are much more evident to patients than to family members, and on their own, are usually not of great importance.

4.1.1.2   Item 2: Body Orientation (Maximum Score 5)

In this test, the integrity of *volitional movements* as well as *right-left orientation* is examined by asking the patient to point to various parts of the body. The right-left disorientation defect shows as inability to carry out instructions which involves an appreciation of right and left. It is a sign of *left cerebral hemisphere dysfunction,* resulting from *dominant* (usually left, in right-handed people) *parietal lobe lesion,* caused by stroke or dementia.

4.1.1.3   Item 3: Praxis (Test for Visuospatial Difficulties, Apraxia and Agnosia)

In order for sensations to be fully appreciated and consciously recognised they have to be perceived, discriminated and associated with existing knowledge. Stimuli have to be processed (appreciation) to form a conscious perception of something. These conscious elements then need to be associated (linked) with other elements (e.g. memory traces) which give them meaning. Abnormality in this higher-level cognitive process leads to *agnosia*, which means non-recognition. It is the failure to appreciate the significance of sensory information in spite of intact sensory pathways and consciousness.

Patients with visuospatial difficulties may make no complaints. Visuospatial agnosia is often associated with constructional dyspraxia. This test has been included to test that. This item tests the patient's ability to carry out purposeful movements to commands. Impairment of praxis is called *dyspraxia* or *apraxia.* Apraxia is the inability to carry out learned, voluntary movement, which cannot be accounted for by paresis, incoordination or sensory loss.

The patient is asked to first observe and learn a set of movements, then asked to repeat them *independently* until you ask them to stop.

4.1.1.4   Item 4: Drawing (Test for Constructional Dyspraxia)

In the original RUDAS the patient is shown a cue card of 'cube drawing' and then asked to draw the picture of the cube on a piece of paper. In the *Nepali* and *Hindi* versions, cube has been replaced with 'stick design test'. The *examiner demonstrates how to arrange four wooden matches as a square shape (Fig. 4.1). The matches are then handed over to the patient to make an exact copy, i.e. align in a square shape.*

Most normal subjects will succeed in copying simple designs. The use of sticks for constructional task gives the opportunity to observe patient's capacity to improve their performance and to alter mistakes.

Scoring
- Is it a four-sided square? (Yes: 1, No: 0)

Does the figure rest on a side? (Yes: 1, No: 0)

Are match heads (Fig. 4.1) correctly oriented? (Yes: 1, No: 0)

4.1.1.5   Item 5: Judgement (Test for Agnosia)

Judgement is an '*Executive Function.* It is the ability to set a goal, initiate and execute it safely avoiding distractions and remaining flexible and responsive to changing circumstances. Patients may lack insight into these issues, but family members tend to be more informative, especially when it comes to cooking and driving.

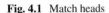

Fig. 4.1 Match heads

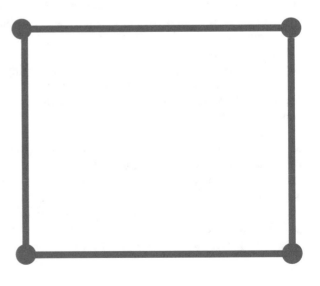

4.1.1.6 Item 1b: Memory (Recall—Max 8 Points)

This test for 'delayed recall' tests episodic memory. *Amnesia* is the name given for acquired memory dysfunction. There is an abnormality in registering, storing, recalling, or recognising information and events. Patients may have deficits in explicit memory, with difficulty on conscious recollection, yet retain implicit (procedural/skills) knowledge. For example, they may be able to find their way around familiar surroundings but be unable to describe their route.

4.1.1.7 Item 6: Language (Animal Naming—Test for Verbal Fluency— Max 8 Points)

Efficient communication of information requires symbols. Language is the ability to code and interpret those symbols. It relates closely to thought.

Abnormality of language is called *dysphasia* (or *aphasia*). Assessing dysphasia is crucial before proceeding with further cognitive testing. There is either a defective understanding (*receptive dysphasia*) or a defective production of speech/writing (*expressive dysphasia*).

Using the telephone is particularly difficult for patients with receptive dysphasia, because all the usual nonverbal cues are absent. Minor expressive speech defects may be noted when the patient is engaged in conversation, during history taking. RUDAS, therefore, does not have separate tests for receptive or expressive aphasia. It uses *verbal fluency* test to assess language function related to frontal lobe lesions. As described in item 6, the simple technique is to ask the patient to name as many animals as he can think in 1 min.

The number of 'animals' named will often be strikingly low even though there is no evidence of aphasia. This is in keeping with the poverty of spontaneous speech which may be observed in frontal lobe lesions. It is necessary to allow the patient a full minute for the test. The effect is more pronounced with left frontal lesions than right.

Total Score

At the end of the test, scores for each item are added up to get a total score out of **30**.

Any score of 22 or less indicates possible cognitive impairment; it can be used as one of the key diagnostic criteria for diagnosing dementia due to Alzheimer's disease.

Please note that the cognitive impairment on its own is not enough to diagnose dementia. Other criteria are also required.

4.2 Screening for Depression

Depression is not a natural part of ageing. In 2020, major depression became the second most burdensome health condition worldwide, taking into account both associated disability and premature mortality. The prevalence of depression rises with age. Late-life depression is a common disorder affecting 10–15% of the elderly population, especially amongst women. Depression is often reversible with prompt recognition and appropriate treatment. However, if left untreated, depression may result in the onset of physical, cognitive, functional, and social impairment, as well as decreased quality of life, delayed recovery from medical illness and surgery, increased health care utilisation and suicide.

Depressive symptoms can be a part of the clinical presentation of dementia, which has led to a debate as to the direction of causation: whether depression is a prodromal symptom or an independent risk factor for dementia. Depression is associated with cognitive impairment in older adults (Box 4.1).

> **Box 4.1 Depression and Dementia (The Framingham Study) [2]**
> In 2010, the famous Framingham Heart study revealed that depression was associated with increased risk of dementia and AD in older men and women over 17 years of follow-up. In 949 Framingham original cohort (mean age = 79) depression, assessed at baseline during 1990–1994, was present in 13.2% of the sample. During the 17-year follow-up period, 164 participants developed dementia; 136 of these cases were AD. *A total of 21.6% participants who were depressed at baseline developed dementia compared with 16.6% of those who were not depressed.* **Depressed participants had more than 50% risk of dementia**. Results were similar when persons with MCI were excluded.

Another cohort study following people for up to 28 years before the development of dementia found that it was only in the 10 years before the onset of dementia that depressive symptoms were higher in people with dementia than those without dementia. This suggests that midlife depression is not a risk factor for dementia. It is biologically plausible that depression increases dementia risk because it affects stress hormones, neuronal growth factors, and hippocampal volume.

There are a number of mechanisms by which depression may impact on the risk of dementia. Chronic inflammatory changes which occur in depression, potentially as a result of stress, may contribute to the development of dementia and AD. Depression may also be associated with vascular factors as described by the vascular depression hypothesis, which postulates that vascular pathology contributes to the pathogenesis of depression in late life. Several life-style factors associated with longstanding depression, such as diet, physical activity, and social engagement, may also increase the risk of dementia. Population-based epidemiological studies have shown that vitamin B12 deficiency and high levels of *homocysteine* are associated with depression in older adults and with an increased risk of dementia and AD.

On the other hand, depression is about twice as common in people with type 2 diabetes compared with those without. Depression and diabetes are risk factors for one another, and both are associated with an increased risk of cognitive impairment. Cognitive impairment in people with type 2 diabetes can result in problems with self-management, treatment adherence and monitoring. It is also known that cognitive impairment often remains unrecognised by physicians. The American Diabetes Association guidelines recommend annual screening for cognitive impairment in older people with diabetes to facilitate patient-centred care aimed at optimising health outcomes and health-related quality of life.

4.2.1 Geriatric Depression Scale (GDS)

While there are many instruments available to measure depression, the Geriatric Depression Scale [3] has been used extensively. The GDS short form (15 questions) has been derived from the original 30-question version. It has been designed for the assessment of depressive symptomatology in elderly and excludes any questions relating to the physical symptoms of depression common in old age. Of the 15 items, 10 questions indicate the presence of depression when answered positively, while the rest (question numbers 1, 5, 7, 11, 13) indicate depression when answered negatively.

The questions (Box 4.2) are *read out* and the patient is asked how they felt over the past week using *Yes/No* response format. No further explanation or interpretation is required. Each answer indicating depression (bold '**yes**' or '**no**') counts for one point. Scores of 0–4 are considered normal; 5–8 indicate mild depression; 9–11 indicate moderate depression; and 12–15 indicate severe depression. *Scores greater than 5 are indicative of probable depression.*

Box 4.2 GDS Short [4]
Instructions: Choose the best answer for how you felt over the past week.

1. Are you basically satisfied with life? Yes/***No***
2. Have you dropped many of your activities and interests? Yes/No
3. Do you feel that your life is empty? Yes/No
4. Do you often get bored? Yes/No
5. Are you in good spirits most of the time? Yes/No
6. Are you afraid that something bad is going to happen to you? Yes/No
7. Do you feel happy most of the time? Yes/No
8. Do you often feel helpless? Yes/No

9. Do you prefer to stay at home, rather than going out and doing new things? Yes/No
10. Do you feel you have more problems with memory than most people? Yes/No
11. Do you think it is wonderful to be alive? Yes/No
12. Do you feel pretty worthless the way you are now? Yes/No
13. Do you feel full of energy? Yes/No
14. Do you feel that your situation is hopeless? Yes/No
15. Do you think that most people are better off than you are? Yes/No

The GDS has a 92% sensitivity and an 89% specificity when evaluated against diagnostic criteria. The GDS is NOT a substitute for a diagnostic interview by mental health professional. It is useful tool in the clinical setting to facilitate assessment of depression in older adults. It does not assess for suicidality. The GDS is in public domain.

References

1. Nepal GM, Shrestha A, Acharya R. Translation and cross-cultural adaptation of the Nepali version of the Rowland universal dementia assessment scale (RUDAS). J Patient Rep Outcomes. 2019;3:38.
2. Saczynski JS, Beiser A, Seshadri S, et al. Depressive symptoms and risk of dementia: the Framingham heart study. Neurology. 2010;75(10):35–41.
3. http://www.stanford.edu/~yesavage/GDS.html
4. Sheikh JI, Yesavage JA. Geriatric Depression Scale (GDS): recent evidence and development of a shorter version. Clin Gerontol. 1986;5(1/2):165–73.

Chapter 5
Diagnosis

*Any clinician who has the appropriate skills can recognise
and make a diagnosis of dementia; and brain scanning is
NOT always needed. Specialist advice may be needed in
particular clinical situations where the presentation or course
is atypical*

Professor Alistair Burns (National Clinical Director of
Dementia, NHS England, 2014)

5.1 Diagnosis of Dementia

Traditionally, medicine is divided into science and art: the 'science' is the body of
medical knowledge and research which inform medicine; the 'art' the process of
diagnosis. Diagnosis is the process of converting the information obtained from history and examination into the names of diseases or syndromes, which, in turn, identify or explain abnormalities in the observed evidence. Thus, diagnosis involves
deductive and inductive logic in order to 'map' symptoms on to a disease. It requires:
(1) an adequate set of disease definitions and classifications; (2) a reasoning process
that will allow the doctor to use the signs exhibited and symptoms expressed by the
patient so as to; (3) make a diagnosis.

The second step of diagnosis is a 'reasoning process'—an orderly process proceeding from the general (the gathering of initial information) to the specific (the
diagnosis). This is where the 'art' of medicine is seen to be located, for much of the
reasoning process is based on the clinician's capacity for inductive logic. Here the
doctor and the patient meet, and the process starts with the doctor attempting to
identify the cause of the illness and ends with applying their clinical judgement in
order to make a diagnosis and arrive at a treatment plan.

Dementia diagnosis may be seen as 'science' which suffers the shortcomings of
not being scientific enough. Alternatively, one may wonder whether dementia

diagnosis *really* an art which is mistakenly apprehended as science? Clinical decision-making has been described as an experiment, where the purpose is to 'repeat a success of the past'. When a laboratory investigator makes decisions in conducting an experiment, we require that the ingredients of his reasoning be explicitly defined. We insist that he be able to specify his methods, his data, and his interpretations of the data, and that the specifications be precise and reproducible. On the other hand, when a clinician makes decisions in the experiment of clinical medicine, we generally assume that the procedure is too complex for scientific documentation. The reasoning process used is quite different from deductive logic, for it, depends not on a knowledge of causes, mechanisms, or names of disease, but on a knowledge of patients. Clinical judgement is therefore an 'art', but as an art it is unproducible in the sense in which experiments are reproducible. The clinician is usually permitted to justify his work, it has been argued, on the basis of 'hunch', intuition, or a nebulously defined clinical experience.

If we look at the human body through Cartesian prism of dualism, the body looks like a machine, and disease as a failure of various mechanical functions. The analogy is made more apt by the process of training of doctors, which seeks to eradicate the expression of emotions, to encourage detachment and to supress signs of 'human weakness'. The metaphor of the medical encounter thus becomes one where one machine is assessed by another, superior, model of machine. The process of dementia diagnosis should perhaps be seen not as the rational, scientific process, but as an interpretative process where the patient seeks to describe his/her symptoms in a language which may only inadequately describe them and the doctor attempts to achieve access to inaccessible signs and symptoms and to transcribe them into a medical terminology which itself is masked by imprecision. *This is doubly so in the case of an older person diagnosed as having Alzheimer's disease as, first, the individual's symptoms are relayed through a third party who can observe only the outer manifestations of this seeming illness, and second, the causes of the disease are not entirely amenable to testing.* Both carers and doctors can thus be seen in the diagnostic encounter as constructing the diagnosis of dementia. No wonder, physicians often do not wish to accord the label of 'Alzheimer's disease', and often are ignorant of the disease.

The diagnosis of dementia is challenging particularly in the early stage as there are no definitive biological markers, the onset is often insidious, and other reversible causes of cognitive impairment either resemble or accompany dementia. Specialists also find some of the components of dementia diagnostic process, especially the disclosure of the diagnosis difficult.

In a questionnaire survey of old age psychiatrists in England (Jha and Walker [1], 2018) for the question '*Which task do you find most difficult in the diagnostic process?*' A relatively large proportion of participants (41%) identified '*discussing driving*' as the most difficult task, followed by '*disclosing diagnosis*' (18%), '*diagnosing subtypes of dementia*' (18%), '*planning post-diagnostic support*' (15%), and '*discussing treatment and prognosis*' (3%). Clinicians spent more time (10–20 min in history taking and cognitive assessment, and less than 10 min in disclosure and discussion of diagnosis. How much time can front-line physicians in developing world spend?

It is commonly held that the principal aim must be to exclude a remedial cause for the patient's symptoms and that the diagnosis of AD is one of exclusion. However, truly reversible causes of dementia are rare in older people. Nor is it true that the diagnosis is one of exclusion. Dementia due to Alzheimer's disease has a characteristic presentation and can be **confidently diagnosed following a careful clinical evaluation**. A full evaluation is important not only to assess the primary disorder but also other concomitant disorders that may be aggravating the situation.

Treatable conditions include cerebral tumour, subdural haematoma, normal pressure hydrocephalus, and certain systemic disorders that may be indirectly impairing cerebral function. These indirect impairments include the several causes of cerebral anoxia, myxoedema, hypoglycaemia, metabolic derangements due to renal or hepatic disease, vitamin deficiencies, alcoholism, and intoxication due to various drugs and chemicals. Occasionally, complete investigation will leave one with probabilities rather than certainties, and it will then be necessary to see what course the disorder takes with time. Lack of clear confirmation of the diagnosis will mean that it is essential to keep the patient under regular review, with readiness to investigate again if necessary.

There is no single 'dementia test'. Cognitive decline, specifically memory loss alone, is not sufficient to diagnose dementia. There needs to an impact on daily functioning related to a decline in the ability to judge, think, plan and organise. There is an associated change in behaviour such as emotional lability, irritability, apathy or coarsening of social skills. There must be evidence of decline over time (months or years rather than days or weeks) to make a diagnosis of dementia. Delirium and depression are the two most common conditions in the differential diagnosis.

The Box 5.1 below provides the DSM-5 criteria for dementia due to Alzheimer's disease.

5.1.1 DSM-5 Criteria for Dementia Due to AD

Box 5.1 DSM-5 Criteria for Probable Major Neurocognitive Disorder Due to Alzheimer's Disease
(a) The (core) criteria are met for major neurocognitive disorder
(b) There is insidious onset and gradual progression of impairment in one or more cognitive domains
(c) **Probable Alzheimer's disease** is diagnosed if either of the following is present:

   1. Evidence of a causative Alzheimer's disease genetic mutation from family history or genetic resting.
   2. **All three** of the following are present: (**a**) clear evidence of decline in memory and learning and at least one other cognitive domain (based on detailed history or neuropsychological testing); (**b**) steadily progressive, gradual decline in cognition, without extended plateaus; (**c**) no evidence of mixed aetiology.

5.1.2 Probable AD Dementia: Core Clinical Criteria

Probable AD dementia is diagnosed when the patient:

1. Meets criteria for all cause dementia, and in addition, has the following characteristics:

    (a) *Insidious onset*. Symptoms have a gradual onset over months to years, not sudden over hours or days;

    (b) Clear-cut *history of worsening* **of cognition** by report or observation; and

    (c) The initial and most prominent cognitive deficits are evident on history and examination in one of the following categories: (a) *amnestic presentation* (impairment in learning and recall of recently learned information; (b)*Non-amnestic presentations:* language presentation, visuospatial presentation or executive dysfunction (impaired reasoning, judgement, and problem solving)

    (d) The diagnosis of probable AD dementia should not be applied when there is evidence of substantial concomitant cerebrovascular disease or core features of other dementias

5.2 Differentia Diagnosis

"Diagnosis of dementia and accurate determination of subtype early in the course of the disease are crucial for optimal clinical care and management."

As discussed earlier on, the diagnosis of Alzheimer's dementia is based on the recognition of the typical syndrome of cognitive improvement affecting patients daily living over a period of time. Atypical presentations should be referred for specialist advice regarding the more unusual sub-types. Vascular dementia in isolation is rare; the majority of presentations are Alzheimer's or mixed dementia, i.e. Alzheimer's and a vascular element.

5.2.1 Differentiating from Normal Ageing

When the process of remembering is slightly slowed, but still intact, we call it 'normal ageing'. By far the most common cause for cognitive change after age 50 is normal ageing of the nervous system. Compared to young adults, older individuals show selective losses in functions related to the *speed and efficiency of information processing*. Particularly vulnerable are memory *retrieval* abilities, *attentional* capacity, *executive skills*, and *divergent thinking*, such as working memory and multitasking.

Unlike the patient with Alzheimer's disease, the older adult without the disease show normal performance on other memory procedures, such as cued recall and delayed recognition. The profile of performance suggests that different mechanisms underlie the memory loss of ageing and Alzheimer's disease. In Alzheimer's, the problem resides in the consolidation or storage of new information in long-term memory stores. In normal ageing, the principal problem is in accessing recently stored information. In normal ageing, the cognitive losses described are annoying but not disabling. In dementia, the difficulties are more pronounced, even in the early stages, leading to functional changes and the need for adjustments in daily life.

5.2.2 *Functional Cognitive Disorder [2]*

The WHO expects every member country to increase the rate of dementia diagnosis. Cognitive symptoms are common, and yet many who seek help for cognitive symptoms neither have, nor go on to develop dementia. A proportion of these people are likely to have functional cognitive disorders- a subtype of functional neurological disorders, in which cognitive symptoms are present, associated with distress or disability, but caused by functional alterations rather than degenerative brain disease or another structural lesion. *Functional memory impairment* or disorder is not an established diagnostic category, but it has been defined as "an acquired medical or psychological condition that is closely related to psychosocial burden and distress".

Increased government and media interest may result in greater number of people seeking help for memory problems. This may not reduce the dementia gap, instead increase numbers seen who do not have dementia. It may also create a risk of false-positive diagnosis, which can have a devastating consequence if incorrectly given. Memory clinic reports have shown an increase in proportion of patients with functional psychiatric disorders (predominantly depression) and also functional memory problems, rather than people with cognitive complaints due to a neurodegenerative dementia.

5.2.3 *Subjective Cognitive Impairment*

An increased public awareness of AD heightens the fear that relatively benign changes in speed of processing and word retrieval are a harbinger of an imminent Alzheimer's disease.

There are some patients who have a strong subjective sense that something is wrong with their memory, but they perform well on objective tests. Many of these patients suffer from chronic depression and/or anxiety—conditions that are, in themselves, significant risk factors for the development of dementia. These patients should be offered pragmatic health advice—especially about exercise, alcohol and vascular risk reduction. Judicious use of antidepressants may be helpful. Patients may benefit from counselling. They may accept an offer of periodic cognitive testing. The person does not need to have a diagnosis of dementia.

5.2.4 Dementia and Delirium

Delirium is perhaps the most common cognitive disorder and a common problem in the differential diagnosis of dementia is mistaking a delirium for dementia. And even more common problem is failing to recognise delirium superimposed on an underlying dementia. Both delirium and dementia manifest as impairment in cognitive functions. The two conditions differ in the pattern of deficits and the cognitive domains that are affected.

In at least the early and middle stages of dementia, the patient is alert and attentive, whereas in delirium the patient shows decreased attention to the environment and has an altered level of arousal. The delirious patient's cognitive deficits fluctuate, whereas those of the patient with dementia are usually stable. In delirium, symptoms should remit once the underlying physiological disturbance is reversed. Recovery from delirium may be delayed in older persons leading to a premature and often mistaken diagnosis of dementia. However, people with dementia are more susceptible to delirium. Delirium can also be subacute or chronic and difficult to distinguish from dementia.

5.2.5 Dementia and Depression

Cognitive impairment due to depressive disorders is distinguished by the patient's self-reported prominent complaints of difficulty with memory and concentration. Apathy, irritability, and reluctance to complete cognitive testing are apparent but without other signs of cognitive impairment.

It is unusual for a major depressive episode to produce such severe cognitive impairment that distinction of the impairment from a specific dementia such as AD is persistently difficult. The clinical examination is helpful in this differential diagnostic problem. The patient with a primary depression is inattentive, excessively aroused (in agitated depression) or lethargic (in retarded depression), poorly motivated during mental state examination, and frequently answers "I don't know" to questions related to cognitive function. Aphasia, apraxia, and anomia are not present in the patients with cognitive symptoms secondary to a primary depression.

The term *depressive pseudodementia* originally implied a misdiagnosis and was introduced to describe cases in which the diagnosis of dementia was changed after remission of cognitive deficits. Depressive pseudodementia might be more accurately classified as *depressive delirium*, given that depression is a manifestation of disrupted brain physiology at the biochemical level; impaired attention and level of arousal are prominent symptoms.

5.2.6 Vascular Dementia

The term 'vascular dementia' literally means a dementia due to vascular disease. It encompasses a group of conditions, including—*multi-infarct dementia, small-vessel disease, post-stroke dementia* and specific *vascular dementia syndrome* (Box 5.2). Pathology of vascular dementia is frequently of a mixed type with diverse presentations in which the loss of brain volume, ventricular enlargement and the cognitive deficits are difficult to distinguish from Alzheimer's disease.

Box 5.2 DSM-5 Diagnostic Criteria for Vascular Neurocognitive Disorder

(a) The criteria are met for major or mild neurocognitive disorder
(b) The clinical features are consistent with a vascular aetiology, as suggested by either of the following:

1. Onset of the cognitive deficits is temporally related to one or more cerebrovascular elements
2. Evidence of decline is prominent in complex attention (including processing sped) and frontal-executive function

(c) There is evidence of the presence of cerebrovascular disease from history, physical examination, and/or neuroimaging considered sufficient to account for the neurocognitive deficits
(d) The symptoms are not better explained by another brain disease or systemic disorder

---

5.2.7 Dementia Due to Parkinson's Disease or Lewy Body Disease

Lewy bodies are the hallmark of the brainstem pathology (especially *substantia nigra*) of Parkinson's disease. In the last 30 years Lewy bodies have been found to occur outside the substantia *nigra* in some patients with late-onset dementia who do not have clinical Parkinson's disease. When Lewy bodies are present diffusely in the cerebral cortex, they cause a specific type of dementia called '*Dementia with Lewy bodies*', or **DLB**. DLB is the third most common dementia after Alzheimer's and vascular dementia. The course is often slightly more rapid than AD.

Cognitive impairment is usually the presenting feature. However, patients may present with parkinsonism or psychosis in the absence of dementia. The classical triad of symptoms of DLB comprises *fluctuating cognitive impairment,*

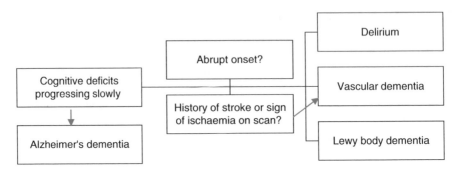

Fig. 5.1 Simplified algorithm for differential diagnosis of dementia

parkinsonism and *visual hallucinations*. The fluctuation may be day to day or even hour to hour and it may be difficult to distinguish from delirium and *Dementia in Parkinson's disease*, which like DLB, also shows considerable fluctuation in attention. Patients with DLB are highly sensitive to extrapyramidal side effects of conventional antipsychotics, especially haloperidol, and should be avoided in treating psychosis in DLB.

Alzheimer's disease, Vascular dementia, and Lewy body dementia make up the vast majority of dementia diagnosis. Figure 5.1 offers a simplified algorithm that will capture 95% of the dementias encountered in memory clinics. The key elements are outlined in Fig. 5.1:

> *Alzheimer's disease, vascular dementia, and DLB make up the vast majority of dementia diagnoses. Figure 5.1 offers a simplified algorithm that will capture 95% of dementias encountered by the average practitioner.*

5.2.8 Misdiagnosis of Alzheimer's

Recent research suggests that patients with Alzheimer's disease who experience psychosis are five times more likely to be diagnosed with Dementia with Lewy Bodies than those without psychosis. Both false positive and false negative rates were 12%.

References

1. https://www.rcpsych.ac.uk/docs/default-source/members/faculties/old-age/old-age-newsletter-jan-18.pdf?sfvrsn=82e1b4ef_2
2. McWhirter L, et al. Functional cognitive disorders: a systematic review. Lancet Psychiatry. 2019;7(2):191–207.

Chapter 6
Supporting Diagnosis and Treatment

> *"As a person with dementia my social health is very important to my daily life. When I was diagnosed social health was never discussed with me. I was much more aware of social disengagement as sadly nobody within the health sector explained to me, I could carry on with my daily life and engagement with my community. I was grieving for life I would never have; I was not offered any post diagnostic support due to my age. I forgot I had rights and should be treated like everyone else and be fully integrated into my community as an equal citizen."*
>
> **Helen Rochford-Brennan** *[1] (Chairperson of the European Working Group of People with Dementia)*

6.1 Support at the Time of Diagnosis

We have deliberately started this chapter with the above quote from a 'Person with dementia', who has written the foreword for an authoritative book, *Timely Psychological Interventions in Dementia Care* [1], written and edited by two acclaimed European dementia specialists.

Doctors are generally well trained in diagnosing and treating diseases, but they are not always trained in how to deliver them properly. People with suspected dementia and their families experience a variety of emotions, worries and concerns at the time of diagnosis and afterward. They need information about their condition, including sensitive discussion about prognosis and limitations of drug treatment. People with dementia need to understand how their cognitive problems affect daily life, and how simple strategies can minimise the impact of these problems and improve their quality of life. People with dementia have to cope with the loss of independence and competence. Support and encouragement are needed to enable them focus on things they can still enjoy and derive a sense of achievement.

A. Jha, K. Mukhopadhaya, *Alzheimer's Disease*,
https://doi.org/10.1007/978-3-030-56739-2_6

Dialogues and conversations with people with dementia regarding these issues are is termed '*psychosocial intervention*'.

In early dementia the principle of psychosocial intervention applies to diagnostic consultation, confidentiality, gaining consent to speak with family members, organising physical investigations, disclosing the diagnosis, starting treatment with drugs, future planning, collaborative care, and more complex decisions such as who should take responsibility when the person with dementia loses the mental capacity to manage property or driving related decisions. Most people with early dementia retain capacity to make decisions in most areas, but families, friends as well as treating physicians often assume otherwise and may sometimes undermine their autonomy. The key to successful psychosocial interventions is that they are individualised to the person and their family tailored to their changing needs.

Historically, mental health services have been vulnerable across the world. In 2008, the Royal College of Psychiatrists launched a 3-year *Fair Deal for Mental Health* [2] campaign to tackle the inequalities faced by people with mental health problems. The College also made a commitment to ensuring that training for psychiatrists promotes the '*Recovery Approach*'. National guidelines emphasised the universal applicability of the recovery values for anyone of any age who has a significant mental health problem. Yet there was little thinking as to whether the recovery approach is applicable to dementia care. Jha et al. [3] in Hertfordshire, UK spotted the striking similarities between a recovery-oriented approach and person-centred care. Through a randomised controlled trial, they have demonstrated that older people's wellbeing and autonomy can be improved by adopting an individualised recovery-oriented approach at routine memory clinics.

The aim of a person-centred recovery approach is to inform and empower the person with dementia and their family to be able to live well with the diagnosis of dementia. This can be achieved by targeting specific goals (established with the person and with their relatives) that can have a concrete impact on people's daily life. Jha et al. have also provided a Mini Wellbeing State Examination (MWeSE) scale [3] specifically for this purpose. We believe that general physician in the developing world can be supported to provide person centred dementia care.

6.2 Disclosure of Diagnosis

Research indicates that patients generally would like to know the diagnosis of dementia [4]. While withholding of diagnosis is distressing for some patients, uncertain and late diagnosis are also unhelpful. The experience of diagnosis disclosure can be distressing for the patient, their family, and also for the doctor. It's like breaking bad news. The person may feel a sense of loss, of stigmatism as well as of hopelessness as a result.

Diagnosis of having Alzheimer's dementia may generate a complex set of emotional states. It is possible to distinguish between primary emotions caused by the experience itself (e.g. loss, grief, rage, fear) and secondary emotions that involve an indirect response to these primary emotions. One of the most significant of these secondary emotions is that of **shame**. *Patients often feel ashamed of being 'weak' or embarrassed of 'displaying one's emotions. These secondary emotions inhibit the emotional processing of the problematic material and which prevent the material being properly assimilated into the existing schema.*

The patient and their family may require time to discuss the diagnosis and its implications. Delivering diagnosis of Alzheimer's disease is a process, not an event. There is a great deal of information to be imparted and the implications of this thought through, and this takes time. The disclosure of diagnosis of dementia should be conducted at least in two interviews, because patients and family may not understand and retain information about the diagnosis after the first interview.

The 'best practice' guidelines for dementia disclosure include preparing for disclosure, integrating family members, exploring the patient's perspective, disclosing the diagnosis, responding to patient reactions, focusing on quality of life and well-being, planning for the future, and communicating all of these sensitively and effectively. As non-specialist doctors you may not have expertise and time to offer that level of care, but you should try to provide alternative sources of information and support. The patient and the family may have the following questions to ask:

Is there any cure?
How long have I got?
What can be done?
Is it hereditary?
Can I still drive?
Will vitamins/crosswords/exercise/diet help?
What about this alternative treatment I've found on the internet?

None of these questions is easy to answer, but you should try to respond honestly and sympathetically. The skills required of professionals in diagnostic disclosure are similar to those used in other serious illnesses such as cancer. A patient-led discussion is preferable with adjustment and compensation for the degree of cognitive impairment and the patients educational and cultural background. Family carers may sometimes attempt to steer their relatives away from diagnostic discussion and it is important to consider whether discussion of the diagnosis should be carried out jointly with a family member or alone with the patient. Following discussion of diagnosis patients should be helped to use the information positively. While discussing treatment, a collaborative approach of decision-making (also known as *shared decision making*) should be adopted. Helping people identify their values is thought to assist them in thinking about, and making, health care choices.

Family carers need to be informed of diagnosis and what to expect in the future. They need to be informed about what services and interventions can help. Sometimes there are problems for carers in balancing their own personal needs with those of the patient. Further difficulties arise where there are pre-existing ambivalent relationships, current ambivalence, and the presence of paranoia (for example leading to accusations or misidentification of the carer).

Box 6.1 provides the **SPIKES** [5] protocol for delivering a diagnosis of Alzheimer's dementia, based on the principles of breaking bad news. SPIKES is an acronym for presenting distressing information in an organised manner to patients and families. The SPIKES protocol provides a six-step framework for difficult discussion:

- Step 1: **S**etting up the interview
- Step 2: Assessing the patient's **P**erception
- Step 3: **I**nviting the patient for further information
- Step 4: Giving **K**nowledge and information to the patient
- Step 5: Addressing the patient's **E**motions with **E**mpathic responses
- Step 6: **S**trategy and **S**ummary

Box 6.1 SPIKES Six-Step Protocol for Delivering Alzheimer's Diagnosis
Mr. Thapa is a 67 old man being seen by a physician at a Kathmandu clinic along with his wife. At the initial assessment, he was found overweight and he was found drinking excessive alcohol. On cognitive testing, he had scored low at **10/30** on RUDAS scale (cut off score **22**). Today, he has come to the clinic to review the findings of the initial assessment with his doctor. He was anxious and worried. Dr. Mishra has been his doctor for a number of years, and he knew that the diagnosis of Alzheimer's will be difficult for him to hear. So, Dr. Mishra sets the stage for this difficult encounter, using SPIKE protocol (acronym for *Setting, Perception, Invitation, Knowledge, Empathy and Strategy*):

1. **Setting:** Before meeting with the patient, Dr. Mishra prepares the setting, the first step of the SPIKES strategy. In preparation of the meeting it is important to review the patient's medical history and facts about the diagnosis prior to his visit. It is important to make sure that the meeting is in a private and a quiet location with enough sitting for everyone present, and set aside enough time for discussion, and minimise distraction, like turning off your mobile phone. Remember to remain calm and attentive.

2. **Perception:** It means, before you tell, ask what the patient knows or expects. In particular how serious he/she thinks the illness is, and/or how much it will affect the future. Verbal (words the patient uses to convey

emotion) and non-verbal (body posture, hand movements) indicate anxiety possibly under a brave front.

Dr. Mishra: *"Tell me how things have been going since we last met"*.

3. **Invitation:** Before you tell, assess how much information the person wants to receive. The real issue is not "Do you want to know?" but "at what level do you want to know?"

Dr. Mishra*: "Let me first explain the result of the memory test, before I tell you what the diagnosis might be"*. Once the patient accepts the invitation to discuss the results, move to the next step of the SPIKES process.

4. **Knowledge:** *In this step, the information is explained.*

Dr. Mishra*: "Your blood tests did not reveal any findings which were new or of concern. Unfortunately, your memory and functioning tests brought some concerns.—Dr Mishra stops for a pause. The patient asks, "What do you mean?"* Dr. Mishra: *"Let me summarise. Your long-term memory is quite good. However, your short-term memory is not so good. That means, remembering words, and difficulty with complex tasks, such as managing money. I wish I had better news Mr and Mrs Thapa. Unfortunately, when we take the results of all the tests together, this suggests a diagnosis of an early stage Alzheimer's disease. That is a most common form of dementia."*

Patient: *"Alzheimer's! At my age! How can that be?"*

Mrs. Thapa*: "Are you sure? Could it be something else? May be medicine he is on?"*

Dr. Mishra: *"Well, I looked at everything. The blood tests, the medication he is on to make sure, I was not missing anything causing your symptoms. Alzheimer's disease is the most likely diagnosis."* The diagnosis is conveyed simply and directly, without any medical jargon. And with empathy. Information is conveyed in small amounts for the patient to process.

5. **Emotion & Empathy:** After reporting the difficult news, address the patient's emotions and show empathy.

Patient: *"My grandmother might have had something like this. I am afraid of getting this"*.

Dr. Mishra: *"I know it is scary, but I am glad you came in and agreed to go through the assessment and examination. The early we know about dementia, the more time we have to plan ahead."*

Mrs Thapa: *"So there is a medicine to cure him."* Dr Mishra: *"No, unfortunately, there is no cure for Alzheimer's at this moment. There are some medications that can slow down how quickly the illness progresses. The purpose of this medication is to help preserve Mr Thapa's memory as much it is possible and for as long as we can."* Mrs Thapa: *"So, what do we do? Start the medication?"*

6. **Strategy**:
   This question leads into planning strategy, which is the last phase of SPIKES. This is where you make sure the patient understands the diagnosis and you collaborate on a plan for the next step. More questions may come. So, provide resources and education. Dr. Mishra: *"It's a good idea to try medicine. I would prescribe a medicine called **donepezil** and we can talk about its risks and benefits. Is it ok with you Mr Thapa?"* After talking about the medicine, Dr. Mishra advised him to cut down the amount of rum and coke, and reduce his weight. He also organised follow-up meetings in 1 and 3 months and handed over a leaflet to Mrs. Thapa containing information about Alzheimer's dementia, prepared by the Alzheimer's Society of Nepal.

It is important for the patient to realise that *"just because they have got a failing memory does not mean they are failing"*. Patients and families need adequate time to discuss the diagnosis and its implications, not only because of the potential emotional impact of the diagnosis, but also because the majority of patients and a significant minority of relatives do not retain information about the diagnosis after the first disclosure. Like some GPs in the UK, you may consider seeing patients with suspected dementia towards the end of your clinic for a longer unhurried period of time.

6.3 Frequently Asked Questions After Diagnosis

Disclosure of diagnosis presents an opportunity to provide patients and families with information about their condition, treatment and sensitive discussion about prognosis. They need to understand how their cognitive problems affect daily life and consider simple strategies to minimise the impact of these problems. They may need to discuss the implication of the diagnosis on driving and related issues. Travel and insurance issues may be discussed along with finance and benefit entitlement. This section discusses some of the frequently asked questions and possible answers and explanations (adapted from case examples from Moniz-Cook et al) [6].

6.3.1 Question 1: Would I End Up in a Nursing Home?

Mrs Brown went to her general physician to discuss her new diagnosis given by the neurologist. She was a 64-year-old store manager in a local grocery shop. She has been complaining problems with her memory and managing the computer system and sales counter. Recently, she experienced difficulty organising 80th birthday party for her husband. She was anxious she might make mistakes at work and so had taken sick leave.

Mrs Brown initially believed she might have a brain tumour although the neurological investigations quickly ruled that out. However, when she received the diagnosis of Alzheimer's disease from the neurologist, she described herself as 'only half prepared'. Her first action was to resign from her job. She wanted to know her diagnosis but felt she had been told in an insensitive way which did not encourage information seeking or offer any hope or reassurance. She had not told either of her daughters or any other friends and family about the diagnosis and was avoiding social contact whenever possible. She had been offered a trial of the anti-dementia drug donepezil but was undecided about this as she felt there was no point. She described an inability to enjoy anything, lack of motivation and a feeling of numbness. She made a new will and drew a power of attorney shortly after hearing the diagnosis.

She had gone to her own physician to discuss the impact of the diagnosis of Alzheimer's disease. She was feeling hopeless and very worried about her future. She experienced frequent intrusive thoughts and imagery of being in a nursing home, highly distressed, and in an advanced state of dementia. She also described feeling of anger and 'why me?' she felt distressed whenever she thought about the diagnosis or was reminded of it in any way.

Her own doctor had special interest in dementia care and listened to her in a way she felt understood. She was helped to understand about her condition and in doing so realised that it could be many years before she reached that level of disability. She had some misinformation stemming from past experience about her husband's memory problems. She felt reassured and agreed to take donepezil as a useful part of her overall coping strategy.

It was suggested that sharing the diagnosis with other family members and close friends could be a good thing, as trying to cover up cognitive problems was exhausting and led to social withdrawal. She was encouraged to pace her activities and not cram too much into one day, to carry out one task at a time and to spend time planning her activities. She was asked to continue activities she knew she could manage, particularly if they were sources of enjoyment. She also recorded activities she was finding difficult and identified what help she would need were she to continue working at the grocery shop. Her daughters were also present at the consultation.

Mrs Brown was gradually able to accept the diagnosis and had more control over her wellbeing. Few months later, she still feared for the future, but these fears were more realistic and less overwhelming. She responded well to the donepezil and intended to continue with it for as long as it proved useful.

Comments: being open with people about diagnosis presents a real opportunity for clinicians. Encouraging patients with dementia share their feelings and asking questions allow us to think and respond more appropriately to the challenges of dementia care. You do not need to be a trained counsellor or a clinical psychologist to offer post diagnostic support. Being sensitive and open are enough to win the trust of the patient and their family.

6.3.2   Question 2: What Are TIAs/Mini Strokes?

Mrs Thakur was a 78-year old housewife who came to the doctor because her husband was convinced that she had dementia and wanted the prescription of Aricept (donepezil) that might help her. Mrs Thakur herself was not interested in any drugs—'let alone drugs for the mind'. She felt that her memory 'was fine'. Mrs and Mr Thakur had used the internet to find out about dementia before attending the clinic. They both agreed that in the past 3 months she had become somewhat hesitant and lacking in confidence, particularly with activities in the home. Mr Thakur felt he now had to do more to assist with preparation of meals and some household tasks. Mrs Thakur had also recently decided to stop driving and discontinue her insurance for their joint car. At the diagnostic assessment, the doctor had discussed the diagnosis of vascular dementia. Mr Thakur remained keen that his wife was offered an anti-dementia drug. Mrs Thakur did not want to take any drug, and having outlined her day-to-day concerns, she requested a second opinion from a renowned neurologist in the nearby city to be sure whether her brain was functioning alright.

The neurologist examined Mrs Thakur and organised a CT scan of her brain. She was told that Transient Ischaemic attacks (TIAs) or 'Mini Strokes' are the second most common cause of memory difficulties in people over 65. They occur when a part of the brain is temporarily deprived of its blood supply, which carries oxygen to the brain. They may occur suddenly and last for quite short periods—between 5 and 30 min and much less in the case of a TIA; others may be aware of 'strange sensations'; and in other cases temporary problems such as double vision, numbness, weakness or tingling in an arm, leg, hand or foot and dizziness are reported. Mostly people feel they have 'recovered' from these episodes after a period of time. Mini strokes can affect any part of the brain—in Mrs Thakur's case they had affected functioning towards the back of her brain. This means that most of the brain was working fairly normally for her age and some parts of the brain may have had taken the function of parts where complete recovery from the mini stroke had not occurred.

6.3.3 Question 3: How Can I Stop Things from Getting Worse?

Mrs Thakur was advised by the doctor to start taking aspirin to thin her blood and thus reduce the likelihood of a further mini stroke. Having high blood pressure can make things worse but her doctor had already prescribed medication for it. She was advised to come to the clinic regularly to monitor her blood pressure at least once a year for blood tests to check that she had not developed new conditions such as pneumonia, diabetes and so on. She was also advised to keep her alcohol intake to a minimum as excessive alcohol, like fat and salt, raise blood pressure. Since she was hypertensive, she was also advised to slightly reduce her caffeine (coffee and tea) intake and eat a well-balanced diet, which is low in fat and salt. Since she was not taking any form of exercise, she was advised to go for a 30-min walk every day.

6.3.4 Question 4: Why Do I Have Trouble 'Getting Going'?

Mrs thakur sometimes had difficulty putting her thoughts into action. Although she knew exactly how to do something and could describe it to others, she had difficulty carrying out the action or activity. She had difficulty starting an activity, i.e. her 'start motor' was slow. Sometimes this can make other people think that she was 'hesitant' or had lost confidence or was being slow, but she was advised to recognise that was not the case. If this occurs, she was told to ask her husband to physically prompt her to get going on a task. Once she gets going, she won't have too much trouble continuing with what she wanted to do.

6.3.5 Question 5: Should I Stop My Social Activities?

It is very important to encourage patients diagnosed with dementia to continue with whatever social activities/hobbies they were doing even though they might be embarrassed at the apparent 'mistakes' they make. Activities like weekly meeting with friends, contact with grandchildren, provide important mental stimulation. They should adopt the policy of 'use it or lose it' and do these activities with people they trust—who will overlook the patients' occasional mistakes and encourage them to get going.

6.3.6 Why Has My Mother Become So 'Lazy'?

A 69-year-old widow has been living with her daughter Kerry for last 20 years. She reported to her doctor that she was concerned about her mother's declining memory. Kerry did not feel that her mother had memory problems but that she had become increasingly 'lazy' and had lost interest in the house. Kerry felt that she had to constantly 'nag' her mother to do things. Both agreed that this had led to increasing tension in the household. When the doctor performed RUDAS cognitive test, the patient had shown signs of 'abnormal executive' functions, what psychologists refer to as **'Dysexecutive Syndrome'**. This syndrome is caused by cognitive deficits in the frontal lobe of the brain causing difficulties with motivation and task initiation. Kerry was able to understand that her mother was not 'lazy'; she was showing signs of early Alzheimer's disease which had affected the front of the brain rather than the temporal lobe which causes memory problems.

6.3.7 Why Does My Husband Not Listen to Me and Avoid Me?

Reduced ability to communicate has an impact on relationships of patients with relatives and treating clinicians. Communication can be affected early on in dementia with *receptive or expressive dysphasia*/aphasia. This may come across as the patient not listening or avoiding conversation. Specific attention to compensating for functional language loss is relevant to everyone involved. Steps taken will include attempting to use a calm and organized environment which is free of distractions; sensory input, both hearing and vision, should be maximized and clear initiation of conversation may be established by use of face-to-face contact or touch; the matters to be discussed should be simplified and presented one at a time. Orientation to the topic of conversation may help, as well as written prompts and reminders. Gesture may remain intact and may be helpful. The person, or those who know them, can help determine in which way they can assist if they get stuck. For example, does sentence completion help or make things worse? Reassurance and support for frustration needs to be given when this occurs.

Dementia contributes to loss of the second language and reversion to mother tongue may confound accuracy of diagnosis. For instance, a Nepalese doctor may find that a patient coming from outside Kathmandu has forgotten to speak in the Nepalese language and reverted back to her native Maithili language. In addition to educational and cultural factors, incorrect assumptions about literacy and misunderstanding of certain concepts can result in overestimating cognitive loss while missing other functional reasons for deterioration in a person's function. Some members of ethnic minority may have been exposed to trauma arising from social upheaval, prior displacement (especially among refugees), and other adverse circumstances that are related to migration. The losses of dementia (in particular loss of control and autonomy) may also trigger the re-emergence of post-traumatic experiences. Recently, during the COVID-19 lock down patients with dementia have been seen to be more irritable and agitated in the face of social distancing and isolation.

6.4 Clinical Management of Early Dementia

The concept of treatable and non-treatable dementias is no longer relevant; all dementias are treatable, albeit not necessarily curable. Disease-modifying therapies are still not available. Cholinesterase inhibitors provide modest stabilisation of changes to cognition and ADLs associated with the disease. They do not reverse or stop the degenerative processes. One of the most effective therapies for AD is proactively managing underlying vascular risk factors.

The core principles of management of early dementia include *improving cognition, maximising independence, maintaining function,* and *planning for the future.* A common point of concern or interest between patient and carer needs to be established with flexibility and sensitivity. Bridges may be built through attention on a physical health focus for some patients while for the carers addressing behavioural and psychological symptoms, such as agitation and sleep disturbances, may be the priority.

6.5 Drug Treatments

Currently, there is no cure for Alzheimer's disease, but there are medicines to help improve symptoms and prevent deterioration. The only approved drug treatments in many countries for cognitive symptoms of dementia are for Alzheimer's disease, dementia with Lewy bodies, or Parkinson's disease dementia. They target biochemical abnormalities as a consequence of neuronal loss, but do not modify the underlying neuropathology or its progression.

Cholinesterase inhibitors are expected to partly restore the deficit in acetylcholine arising from loss of neurones in the nucleus basalis of Meynert (see Box 6.2), and in the central septal area, projecting to cortical regions. The search for abnormalities in brain neurotransmitter system in Alzheimer's disease was inspired by the successful use of L-dopa in treating dopamine deficiency in Parkinson's disease.

Box 6.2 Alzheimer's Eureka Moments

In the late 1970s, a deficit in the brain presynaptic cholinergic system was discovered in post-mortem brain tissues from patients with AD. This cholinergic deficiency hypothesis was confirmed in 1982 when scientists discovered extensive neuronal loss in the cholinergic nucleus basalis of Meynert in patients with AD. This basal forebrain structure is the primary source of cholinergic projection to the neocortex and hippocampus.

Another important discovery was that acetylcholinesterase inhibitors (AChE), which increase intrasynaptic acetylcholine levels, produce modest symptomatic improvement and slow symptomatic deterioration. Inhibition of AChE prevents the breakdown of acetylcholine Tacrine was the first cholinesterase inhibitor demonstrated to be effective in AD in 1994. However, tacrine was abandoned due to liver toxicity, and replaced by second-generation cholinesterase inhibitors (e.g., donepezil), which are equally effective.

The severity of dementia in Alzheimer's disease correlates with the number of neurofibrillary tangles in the brain. Under electron microscope, these tangles are seen as 'paired helical filaments', long fibrous proteins braided together like strands of a rope. These filaments consist of the microtubule-associated protein tau, which normally functions as a bridge between the microtubules in axons, ensuring that they run straight and parallel to one another. In Alzheimer's disease, the tau detaches from the microtubules and accumulates in the soma. This disruption of the cytoskeleton causes the axon to die, thus hampering the normal flow of information in the affected neurones. What causes such changes in tau?

Scientists are working on another protein that accumulates in the brain of Alzheimer's patients, called amyloid. The consensus today is that the 'abnormal secretion of amyloid by neurones is the first step in the process that leads to neurofibrillary tangle formation and dementia'—the amyloid cascade theory. The newest focus of drug research is for the drug to reduce or prevent the depositions of amyloid in the brain.

These drugs have similar efficacy in improving symptoms of cognition, function and behaviour. They may also delay the onset of the behavioural and psychological symptoms found in more advanced stages of dementia, reduce caregiver burden, and delay care home placement. As there is no means of determining who will, or will not, respond to these anti-dementia drugs, we usually prescribe for a 3-month trial of efficacy with gradual increase of the dose. Side effects tend to appear mostly during the initial, titration phase of treatment. Adverse events tend to be short-lived. A great majority of patients experience only minimal side effects, the number of patients discontinuing treatment because of adverse events is fewer in clinical practice than in the clinical trials. However, caution should be exercised in patients with cardiac conduction defects or significant bradycardia.

Caution: *Ideally, acetylcholinesterase inhibitors should only be prescribed in settings where the specific diagnosis of Alzheimer's disease can be made **and** where adequate support and supervision by specialists is available. However, physicians prepared to review adherence, dosing and improvement may consider prescribing if carers are available to monitor side effects and adherence. It is important to bear in mind that even if no medications are prescribed, **there is much that can be done** to improve the quality of life of the person with dementia and their carers.*

6.6 Cholinersterase Inhibitors (Appendix B)

Three cholinesterase inhibitors, donepezil, rivastigmine, and galantamine, are in routine use.

6.6.1 Donepezil

Donepezil was licenced in Europe in 1997 as the first available treatment for mild to moderately severe AD. *Donepezil* is available as tablet or orodispersible tablet; *rivastigmine* is available as a transdermal patch or capsule or liquid, and *galantamine* as a capsule.

One of the early pivotal studies evaluated the use of donepezil at either 5 mg or 10 mg against placebo, over a 6-month period, in 473 patients. A quarter of patients taking the higher, 10 mg, dose improved by gaining 6–12 months' gain in cognitive function compared with their baseline level. Further studies have found the efficacy of donepezil up to 240 weeks.

Although a large majority of patients respond well to donepezil group of drugs, not all of them show similar improvement. There is no means of determining who will, or will not, respond to such treatment, 3–6 months treatment trial with an AChE is recommended.

The beneficial cognitive effects of higher dose of donepezil are mirrored by the adverse event profile, especially gastrointestinal side effects. Fortunately, these side effects are usually short-lived, and majority are free of adverse effects, or experience only minimal symptoms.

Caution should be exercised in those patients with conduction defects as these drugs may cause severe **bradycardia**. Therefore, donepezil group of drugs is contraindicated in heart block or pulse rate below 50/min.

6.6.2   Memantine

Memantine is a non-competitive modulator of the N-methyl-D-aspartate receptor and normalises *glutamatergic neurotransmission*. It prevents excitatory aminoacid neurotoxicity, and is the only drug licenced for severe Alzheimer's disease. It is usually given up to a dose of 20 mg per day.

A combination of memantine and cholinesterase inhibitor has recently been recommended for moderate-to-severe AD.

6.6.3   Souvenaid

Souvenaid is a medical food product for oral consumption formulated to meet nutritional requirements in Alzheimer's disease. It comprises of several ingredients that are hypothesised to be useful as precursors and cofactors for the formation of neuronal membranes, and consumption of souvenaid increases their concentrations.

6.7   Herbal Cholinesterase Inhibitors

In addition to the cholinesterase inhibitors and memantine, researchers have studied herbal medications, *huperzine* and *bacopa* to treat cognitive symptoms of AD.

Huperzine [7], is a Chinese herb extract, which may have some beneficial effects on patients with AD.

Similarly, Mishra et al. [8] have recently reported the preliminary findings of positive response of **Brahmi (Bacopa monnieri Linn)** on patients with dementia. *Brahmi* is an over the counter widely available Ayurvedic herb traditionally used in India as a memory-enhancer.

However, the findings of these studies should be interpreted with caution due to the preliminary nature of the reported studies.

6.8   Immunotherapy with Aducanumab

In October 2019, the pharmaceutical company, Biogen announced that the anti-amyloid antibody *aducanumab* has shown modest but significant efficacy in a phase 3 trial, providing important validation of amyloid A β hypothesis of Alzheimer's disease. *Aducanumab* is a human monoclonal antibody that selectively binds to amyloid β fibrils and soluble oligomers.

Recent research has focused on therapies targeting amyloid precursor protein metabolism, A β_{1-42} deposition or clearance. For example, inhibition of the enzymes β-secretase, which is responsible for the metabolism of amyloid precursor protein.

Two types of immunotherapies are under investigation—injecting amyloid to create host immunity (*active immunization*) and injecting intravenous immunoglobin antibodies to clear amyloid from the brain (*passive immunization*). *Aducanumab* is an example of passive immunization, by binding with soluble Aβ and promoting its removal from the brain through the blood stream.

6.9   Summary Drug Treatment and the Future

Cholinesterase inhibitors (donepezil, rivastigmine, and galantamine) have small but clinically important effect on cognition and function (of all severities of) in Alzheimer's disease but have side effects. Memantine has a smaller effect on cognition, but useful for people who cannot tolerate the side effects of cholinesterase inhibitors. Disease-modifying therapies, including passive immunization, are under investigation.

6.10   Other Cognitive Interventions

Cognitive stimulation therapy [9] has recently been found to improve cognition. It is a group-based therapy led by a trained coordinator incorporating social activity, reminiscence, and simple cognitive exercises (Box 6.3).

Box 6.3 Cognitive Stimulation Therapy (CST)
The aim of CST is to actively mentally stimulate participants through cognitive activities and reminiscence, multisensory stimulation, and group social contact. Each session is let by a facilitator. The standard CST model is a group intervention of 14 themed sessions, each lasting approximately 45 min and held twice per week. This standard programme has been manualised and can be potentially administered by anyone working with people with dementia and held in care homes, hospitals, or day centres.

The programme includes:

- *A non-cognitive warm-up activity (e.g. soft ball game and song)*
- *Elements of really orientation including a board displaying personal and orientation information*

Sessions then focus on different themes, including childhood, food, current affairs, use of money, faces, scenes, and quizzes or word games.

6.11   Specific Management Issues

6.11.1   Planning for the Future

At an early stage of Alzheimer's, patients usually still have the capacity to make decisions about their care in the future and should be actively involved in decision-making. They may be aware that they are beginning to find it difficult to manage their financial affairs, perhaps forgetting how much money they have withdrawn from the bank. It is important to discuss whom they would like to nominate for managing their financial affairs when they are no longer able. They may become vulnerable to financial exploitation. They may also wish to legally appoint someone to make decisions about their future health and social care. Using the relevant laws and regulations of the country of residence, people with early dementia may be able to make advance decisions about life-sustaining treatment. These decisions need to be made after considerable thought and discussions between patients and family members.

6.11.2   Maximising Communication

Communication can be affected early on in dementia with receptive or expressive aphasia. The pragmatics of language (turn-taking and topic management) may also be affected. Reduced ability to communicate has an impact on relationships as well as on the wellbeing of the patient. Family members should be encouraged to use clear, simple conversation, to reduce high emotional expression, use memory aids, and to be non-judgemental.

Specific attention to compensating for functional language loss is relevant to everyone involved. Steps taken will involve:

- *Attempting to use a calm and organized environment which is free of distractions*
- *Sensory input, both hearing and vision, should be maximized and clear initiation of conversation may be established by use of face-to-face contact or touch*
- *The matters to be discussed should be simplified and presented one idea at a time*
- *Orientation to the topic of conversation may help, as well as written prompts and reminders*
- *Gestures may remain intact and may be helpful*

The person, or those who know him or her well, can help determine in which way they can be assisted with if they get stuck. For example, does sentence completion help or make things worse. Reassurance and support for frustration needs to be given when this occurs.

Validation therapy is an approach to communication which acknowledges and supports the feelings of a disorientated person in whatever reality they experience rather than grounding them in the here and now.

6.11.3 Maintaining Function Through Pleasurable Activities

Loss of opportunities to engage in pleasurable and rewarding activities is important both for the individual and for carers since such losses contribute to a vicious cycle of reduced communication, lower mood, less participation in any activity, and increased dependence on others.

As the disease progresses there needs to be an on-going process of finding activities within the person's ability, and structured approach can be helpful. Carers who are aware of appropriate and enjoyable activities enjoy an improved sense of satisfaction and reduced feelings of burden.

There may also be a preventive role; for example, at day centres or social clubs the combination of structured exercises and conversation may reduce deterioration in mobility.

6.11.4 Caring the Carers

It is worth keeping in the mind that the diagnosis of dementia also has important implications for primary carers—the person closest to the patient (usually the spouse), who suddenly finds themselves wearing the label 'carer or *caregiver*' and often need support themselves. Thus, dementia care is not simply a reaction to a crisis; it also involves enabling caregivers to continue caring for an indefinite and often uncertain periods of time. They require psychosocial support in forms of active listening and emotional support.

Physicians may want to do something to help families but may not know what to do. There is some evidence that providing knowledge and opportunity for the families to access the right help for a particular problem during problem through solving consultations may be effective. Goals may be broken down into small clear and achievable entities. For example, physicians may be able to assist the carer to get a good night's sleep by prescribing a hypnotic for them. Research suggests that even when only small and limited goals are achieved, an unbearable situation may change into one where there is still some hope and pleasure in life. Family carers can be empowered to realise their wishes and avoid things that they do not wish to do. Through this process of mobilising caregivers' strengths, there is a possibility that exhaustion or burnout may be prevented.

The provision of both practical and emotional support to patients and their families is critical at all stages of their journey. Caring for persons with advanced dementia is extremely demanding. Without support, caregivers feel exhausted, isolated, and unable to cope. Since specialist dementia care services are not available in developing countries, onus of care falls on the immediate family and relatives. As the local physicians, you may be able to mobilise local community resources to set up day care, sitting services, along with transport and shopping for the affected families.

6.11.5   Management of Neuropsychiatric Symptoms

Neuropsychiatric symptoms in dementia are common; they generally increase with severity of dementia and affect nearly everyone with dementia at some point during their illness. Although many different symptoms exist, they often co-occur in clusters—affective, psychotic, and other symptom clusters. They also vary with the underlying cause of dementia, with visual hallucinations being more common in Lewy body dementia.

Distressing problems arising with progression of dementia include sleep disturbance, behavioural problems, such as agitation, wandering, swallowing difficulties, incontinence, and immobility. Behavioural and psychological symptoms (BPSD) are summarised in Table 6.1:

The overlap between these symptoms highlights the need for careful assessment of symptoms and potential causes, advocated by the DICE (Box 6.4).

Box 6.4 DICE Approach to Manage BPSD
- *Describe the problem*
- *Investigate the cause*
- *Create a plan*
- *Evaluate the effectiveness of it*

6.11.5.1   Depression

People with early dementia may have comorbid depressive illness. The prevalence of depression in dementia is around 20%. They exhibit typical symptoms of

Table 6.1 Behavioural and psychological symptoms of dementia

Behavioural symptoms	Psychological symptoms
• Night-time disturbances • Wandering • Agitation • Aggression	• Anxiety • Hallucinations • Delusions • Uncontrollable emotional outbursts

depression including *anhedonia* (lack of pleasure in life), *amotivation, tearfulness, insomnia,* and *lack of appetite.*

> *As effective treatment often improves cognition and function, a new diagnosis of dementia should usually be suspended until after the depressive illness is successfully treated.*

Treatment of depression in early dementia is likely to enhance psychological wellbeing, physical function (through improved motivation, and general quality of life. Older patients often tolerate tricyclic antidepressants with fewer anticholinergic side effects (e.g. lofepramine) or an SSRI. Possible side effects include gastrointestinal bleeding, hyponatraemia, and falls and fractures.

6.11.5.2 Agitation

Agitation constitutes a range of behaviours, including restlessness, pacing, repetitive vocalisations, and verbal and physical aggression. The behaviours are often accompanied by a feeling of inner tension, although this tension is more difficult to detect in people with advanced dementia.

The cause of agitative symptoms varies. They might be a communication of physical or psychological distress, a misinterpretation of threat, or result from delusions or hallucinations in a person with dementing disease, which reduces their ability to communicate, satisfy, or even know their needs. Agitated behaviours are more common in moderate or severe dementia, especially in care homes, because the symptoms are associated with the breakdown of care in domestic settings leading to care home admission. This makes caring for people with dementia more difficult and time consuming.

Management of Agitation

Management of agitation in dementia should start with asking the person what is wrong. If they cannot articulate or communicate, the following causes of agitation should be considered and addressed, whether the person is feeling:

- Frightened
- Hungry
- Thirsty
- Hot or cold
- In pain

Overstimulation or complex environments might also exacerbate agitation. Interventions to manage agitation and aggression primarily depends on improving caregivers' attitude and communication skills. Caregivers need to have time and patience to identify and respond to the person's wishes in the spirit of so called 'person-centred care'.

6.12 Psychosocial Interventions

From a social perspective, dementia can be viewed as one of the ways in which an individual's personal and social capacities may change for a variety of reasons.

A psychosocial approach should:

- Focus on retaining abilities and avoiding negative stereotyping;
- Provide activities that promote autonomy;
- Normalise or personalise activity support by basing this on knowledge of patients' past pleasure, values and interests; and
- Provide a gatekeeping function to prevent others—such as families and professionals—from undermining access to interventions by the person with dementia,

The management protocol of the WHO mhGAP intervention Guide recommends the use of psychosocial interventions comprising of the following components:

1. Psychoeducation
2. Management of behavioural and psychological symptoms
3. Promotion of functioning in activities of daily living and community life and
4. Interventions to improve cognitive functioning

6.12.1 Follow-Up

It is important to remember that dementia is a progressive and degenerative disorder. There will be deterioration in the person's cognitive, emotional, behavioural and physical functioning along with their ability to carry out the activities of daily living. People diagnosed with AD should be reviewed at least every 3 months.

If not on medications, initiate pharmacological intervention, if appropriate.

If on medication, review adherence, side effects and dosing. Adjust or consider alternative medication as appropriate.

In addition, review psychosocial interventions and evaluate for medical problems.

Assess safety risks and offer appropriate behaviour modification if disease has progressed (e.g. limit driving, cooking, etc.)

Assess for new BPSD, symptoms of depression and risk of self-harm.

Continue assessing carer's needs and provide psychosocial support to both patients and carers throughout their dementia journey, including end of life care.

References

1. Rochford-Brennan H. Foreword. In: Manthorpe J, Moniz-Cook E, editors. Timely psychosocial interventions in dementia care: evidence-based practice. London: Jessica Kingsley Publishers; 2020.
2. Deahl MP. The Fair Deal campaign: a call to arms. Br J Psychiatry. 2010;197(1):1–2.
3. Jha A, Jan F, Gale T, et al. Effectiveness of a recovery-orientated psychiatric intervention package on the wellbeing of people with early dementia: a preliminary trial. Int J Geriatr Psychiatry. 2013;28(6):589–96.
4. Jha A, Tabet N, Orrell M. To tell or not to tell—comparison of older patients' reaction to their diagnosis of dementia and depression. Int J Geriatr Psychiatry. 2001;16(9):879–85.
5. Baile WF, Buckman R, Lenzi R, et al. SPIKES—a six-step protocol for delivering bad news: application to the patient with cancer. Oncologist. 2000;5:302–11.
6. Moniz-Cook E, Gibson G, Harrison J, et al. Timely psychosocial interventions in a memory clinic. In: Moniz-Cook E, Manthorpe J, editors. Early psychosocial interventions in dementia: evidence-based practice. London: Jessica Kingsley; 2009. p. 60–2.
7. Yang G, Wang Y, Tian J, et al. Huperzine A for Alzheimer's disease: a systematic review and meta-analysis of randomized clinical trials. PLoS One. 2013;8(9):e74916.
8. Mishra M, et al. Brahmi (Bacopa monnieri Linn) in the treatment of dementias—a pilot study. Future Healthc J. 2019;6(Suppl 1):69.
9. Spector A, Thorgrimsen L, Woods B, et al. Efficacy of an evidence based cognitive stimulation therapy programme for people with dementia: randomised controlled trial. Br J Psychiatry. 2003;183:248–54.

Appendix A: RUDAS

Rowland Universal Dementia Assessment Scale
(Storey, Rowland, Basic, Comfort & Dickson, 2004). International Psychogeriatrics, 16 (1), 13–31

Date: _____/____/____   **Patient Name:** _____

RUDAS ITEM	Max Score

MEMORY

1. (Instructions) *I want you to imagine that we are going shopping. Here is a list of grocery items. I would like you to remember the following items which we need to get from the shop. When we get to the shop in about 5 minutes' time I will ask you what it is that we have to buy. You must remember the list for me.*

Tea, Cooking oil, Egg, Soap

Please repeat this list for me (ask the person to repeat the list 3 times). (If the person did not repeat all four words, repeat the list until the person has learned them and can repe at them, or, up to a maximum of five times.)

VISUOSPATIAL ORIENTATION

2. *I am going to ask you to identify/show me different parts of the body.* (Correct = 1). Once the person correctly answers 5 parts of this question, do not continue as the maximum score is 5.

1. *Show me your right foot*

2. *Show me your left hand*

3. *With your right hand touch your left shoulder*

4. *With your left hand touch your right year*

5. *Which is (*indicate/point to) *my left knee*

6. *Which is* (indicate/point to) *my right elbow*

7. *With your right hand   indicate/point to my left eye*

8. *With your left hand indicate/point to my left foot*

PRAXIS

3. *I am going to show you an action/exercise with my hands. I want you to watch me and copy what I do. Copy me when I do this …* (One hand in fist, the other palm down on the table – alternate simultaneously.) *Now do it with me: Now I*

*Any score of **22 or less** suggests possible cognitive impairment requiring full dementia assessment.*

Appendix B: Medicine Information (Cholinesterase Inhibitors)

Following the prescription of anti-Alzheimer's drugs, patients and families should be given a written copy of 'Medicine Information' sheet about the medicine. The NHS Medicines Information (A and B) may be translated into local language.

Box A: Acetylcholinesterase Inhibitors
(Pronounced: **a-see-tile-col-in-ester-ase**)

What are acetylcholinesterase inhibitors used for?

Acetylcholinesterase (AChE) inhibitors are usually used to help treat symptoms of dementia specifically caused by Alzheimer's disease. Examples of AChE inhibitors are donepezil, galantamine and rivastigmine. Your medicine may also have a trade or brand name. This is the name that the manufacturer gives to the medicine, for example Aricept® is a brand name for donepezil.

What are the benefits of taking AChE?

People with dementia may have a range of symptoms, which affect the memory, behaviour and the ability to carry out normal daily activities. These activities may include taking care of personal hygiene and nutrition as well as communicating with other people. People may become anxious and their mood and confidence can be affected.

AChE inhibitors do not cure Alzheimer's disease but can help to treat some of these symptoms and keep them under control in the longer term. They may also temporarily slow down the progression of the illness.

© The Editor(s) (if applicable) and The Author(s), under exclusive license to Springer Nature Switzerland AG 2021
A. Jha, K. Mukhopadhaya, *Alzheimer's Disease*,
https://doi.org/10.1007/978-3-030-56739-2

How quickly do AChE inhibitors work?

It may take a period of weeks for AChE inhibitors to have their full effect, some symptoms may start to improve before others. Not everybody benefits from AChE inhibitors, but most people do. If you do not feel any benefit after 4–6 weeks, you should discuss this with your doctor or healthcare worker.

What are the usual doses of AChE inhibitors and how should I take them?

AChE inhibitors are usually started at low doses that are gradually increased, depending on how you respond to the treatment.
The usual dose of donepezil is between 5 milligrams (mg) and 10 mg once a day. The maximum dose is 10 mg once a day. It is usually taken as a single dose (best at bed time).
Do not change your dose without checking with your doctor, as it can affect your response to the medication or may be harmful.

What should I do if I miss a dose?

You will get the most out of your medication when taken correctly and regularly. If you miss or forget a dose at your usual time, but remember within an hour or two take it straight away. If it is longer than this just leave out the missed dose and take the next dose at the usual time. Never take extra medication at the next dose. If you find it difficult to remember taking medication speak to your pharmacist or healthcare worker.

For how long should take *AChE inhibitors?*

Your doctor will discuss with you the length of treatment. It may be for a few months or longer. Your doctor should regularly review your medication to make sure that you do not take medicines for longer than needed. AChE inhibitors are not addictive.

What are the side effects of AChE inhibitors?

As with all medicines there is a risk of unwanted effects (side effects). Some can occur soon after starting treatment so you may experience these before you feel better. Most are temporary and should go away after a few days or weeks. Not everyone will get side effects and many people experience them to different degrees. If you feel that you have side effects that are causing you discomfort, discuss this with your doctor, pharmacist, nurse, or healthcare worker. The table on the following page lists some of the main recognised side effects.

What about alcohol?

Both alcohol and AChE inhibitors? Can affect the brain so it is not recommended that you drink alcohol while taking AChE inhibitors. Drinking alcohol can cause drowsiness, especially heavy drinking. Once you are used to the medication and know the effects of taking alcohol you may be able to drink alcohol occasionally and in small amounts. It is good to be cautious because alcohol affects people in different ways, especially when taking medication.

Do not stop taking your medication because you feel like drinking alcohol. If you drink alcohol, drink only small amounts. Never drink alcohol and drive while taking medication.

What about other medicines?

If you take any other medicines or herbal remedies including any that have been newly prescribed or bought, it is important to check with your doctor or pharmacist that they are safe with AChE inhibitors.

When I should be cautious?

It is usually safe to take AChE inhibitors regularly, as prescribed by your doctor, but they are not suitable for everyone. If any of the following situation apply to you, you should tell your doctor immediately:

- *If you are allergic to AChE inhibitors (if you have taken one before and developed a rash, itching, swollen mouth or throat);*

- *If you have epilepsy (or have had a fit in the past), suffer from kidney or liver disease, heart problems or have asthma or any other long-term lung disease;*
- *If you have difficulty passing urine or have an enlarged prostate;*
- *If you have had stomach or duodenal ulcer;*
- *If you are going to have an operation that requires you to have general anaesthesia you should inform your doctor and anaesthetist that you are taking an AChE inhibitor;*

1.1.1 Side Effects

Side effects	What is it, and what should I do if it happens to me?
Abdominal pain	*Pain in the stomach area*, is most common at the start of the treatment. It should settle after a couple of weeks. If this continues or gets worse, speak to your doctor at your next appointment.
Anxiety or agitation	If you feel *tense, fearful or on edge*, try relaxation methods. Speak to your doctor over the next few days.
Confusion	*Unclear thoughts*
Diarrhoea	*Loose bowel motion* is most common at the start of the treatment. It should settle after a couple of weeks. If this continues, or gets worse, inform the doctor
Dizziness	If you feel *light-headed or faint*, do not stand up quickly. Try and lie down when you feel dizzy. Do not drive.
Drowsiness	If you feel *sleepy or sluggish*, do not drive or use machinery. This is most common at the start of the treatment, and if your medicine is taken once a day it may help to take it at bedtime.
Headache	If your is pounding or painful, try a mild painkiller such as paracetamol.
Loss of appetite and weight loss	If you start eating less and losing weight, speak to your doctor at your next appointment.
Nausea, vomiting	*Feeling and being sick* is the most common side effect at the start of treatment, and usually subside after a couple of weeks.
Tremor	If you feel *shaky* or *stiff*, your doctor may change your medication to one that is less likely to cause tremors.
Rashes and pruritus	Sometime some people develop red rashes on skin, which are itchy. Contact your doctor over the next few days.
Urinary incontinence	If you experience *leakage of urine from the bladder,* it may be just a few drops or a dribble, or may be a stream, speak to your doctor at the next appointment.
Bradycardia (uncommon: one in 100)	If you experience *slowing of the heartbeat,* speak to your doctor as soon as possible. *AChE inhibitors should not be taken if pulse rate is below **50/ min**. Your doctor may reduce the dose or change to a different class of medicine.*

Seizures (**Rare***: one in 1000–10,000 people taking this medicine may get this side effect*)
If you have a *fit, attack, turn or blackout*, contact your doctor immediately.

Index

Printed in the United States
by Baker & Taylor Publisher Services